A Fine Line

George C. Dertadian

A Fine Line

Painkillers and Pleasure in the Age of Anxiety

palgrave
macmillan

George C. Dertadian
School of Social Sciences
University of New South Wales
Kensington, NSW, Australia

ISBN 978-981-13-1974-7 ISBN 978-981-13-1975-4 (eBook)
https://doi.org/10.1007/978-981-13-1975-4

Library of Congress Control Number: 2018950494

Cover image: Ziviani

This Palgrave Macmillan imprint is published by the registered company Springer Nature Singapore Pte Ltd.
The registered company address is: 152 Beach Road, #21-01/04 Gateway East, Singapore 189721, Singapore

Foreword

At times of public health crisis, our attention is justifiably gripped by the most devastating effects and extreme forms of suffering. We are in the midst of what media commentators describe as a deadly epidemic of 'killer' drugs. More accurately, we face an escalation and intensification of harm associated with drug use. Rates of opiate use, especially prescription pain medications, have risen sharply. Overdose deaths are at unprecedented levels. People are struggling with the consequences of their opiate use, consequences which are exacerbated and, in more than a few cases, caused by the effects of prohibitionist and punitive drug policies. In North America, the powerful synthetic opioid Fentanyl has contaminated the illicit drug supply, producing dramatic increases in risk and harm. The US Centers for Disease Control and Prevention have described this as the worst drug overdose epidemic in history.

In this historical moment, it is easy to overlook the reality that the majority of people who use opiates do not develop such dramatic problems and are not represented in medical statistics. This is the case whether their consumption is medically authorised or not. More broadly, the use of analgesic drugs, both prescribed and purchased over the counter, is a part of ordinary life for ordinary people. *A Fine Line* is timely and compelling because it explores the consumption practices of such people, placing their use in the context of the challenges they negotiate, the feelings they seek and the opportunities they desire. In *A Fine Line* we read of painkillers helping men and women to contribute to family life despite chronic pain, to cope with emotional distress, to enhance productivity, to 'chill out' after a night of partying, and to save money by enhancing the effects of alcohol. While not denying the potential harms of routine analgesic use (including dependence), Dertadian eschews sensationalism and moral stances in his presentation of a range of pharmaceutically mediated practices. Crucially these practices include the pursuit of pleasure. *A Fine Line* is therefore an insightful contribution to the sociological literature on pharmaceuticalization, the process by which medical drugs are constituted as the solution for an increasing range of problems and conditions (Fox and Ward 2008). However, Dertadian carefully attends to the heterogeneous experiences of users rather than adopting a predetermined critical narrative. He resists the constitution of medicalization and pharmaceuticalization as singular and monolithic processes.

The large and rapidly growing body of literature on prescription opiate use is primarily epidemiological or clinical, highlighting disease and disorder at either population or individual level. What is missing is the dynamic social environment and the network of relationships in which drug use actually takes place. The epidemiological research which produces the most authoritative 'objective' information on drug use patterns and effects is necessarily abstract, isolating 'factors' from their context in order to identify causal relationships at a population level. As Steve Wing has observed, the 'populations' of modern epidemiology are conceptualised as vehicles for statistical analysis rather than groups with unique histories involving economic, social and ecological relationships (1994). At the same time, epidemiology reduces features such as gender, class and relationship status to individual attributes. In contrast, the accounts of everyday painkiller use collected in *A Fine Line* are based on conversational in-depth interviews with users, carried out by the author. The book exemplifies the rich, detailed and empathetic knowledge of social practices that can be produced by well-executed qualitative research. This research reveals not just what people do but how they make sense of their actions and what meanings they attach to their experiences over time.

The special value of *A Fine Line* resides in its combination of empirical research with recent scholarship in critical drug studies. Theoretical and conceptual examination of dominant approaches to substances and substance use translates the evidence provided by lived experience into a coherent argument about the regulatory effects of medico-legal structures. One of the most important messages of *A Fine Line* concerns the categories we use to understand and respond to complex phenomena such as pharmaceutical consumption. 'Non-medical use' has become the standard term to refer to the consumption of prescription drugs in ways that are not medically authorised, for example for 'non-therapeutic purposes' or 'without a valid prescription'. The abbreviation NMUPD reflects the reification of this classificatory framework and the problem of illegitimate consumption it constructs. Dertadian's analysis highlights both the regulatory function of the category 'non-medical' and its instability. As he points out, patients with chronic pain seek out analgesics for the feeling of relief, which is difficult to demarcate from a positive experience of pleasure, although the latter is labelled as 'non-therapeutic' and therefore suspect. He also points out how medical and legal discourse constitutes the sharing of drugs through a lens of 'non-adherence' and 'diversion', ignoring the elements of care that are expressed through informal networks of distribution.

By placing twenty-first century painkiller use in a historical context, *A Fine Line* reveals another effect of medical authority. Concentrating on the risks of users' unauthorised and non-compliant consumption of medications can act to distract attention from iatrogenic harms. In the current opiate crisis, the actions of Purdue Pharma and the prescription practices of physicians have come under the spotlight, but this has not undermined the confident assertion of a clear distinction between medical (beneficial) and non-medical (harmful) use. Alongside contemporary analgesia, Dertadian includes an instructive discussion of the popularity of over-the-counter headache powders such as Bex and Vincents in Australia in the 1950s. These accessible medications included a combination of aspirin, phenacetin and caffeine (APC). High levels of use produced a sharp increase in gastric ulceration and kidney failure, especially among women. However, as Dertadian notes, there was reluctance among the medical profession to connect normalised and domesticated use of a 'safe' medication with severe harm. He also notes that 'the circumstances of women's lives were left out of the equation in medical accounts of APC consumption'. The repetition of this form of exclusion continues to limit responses to drug use risks and harms.

Despite its critical perspective on medical power, *A Fine Line* does not imagine or hope for a space of freedom, nature or authenticity where individuals live their lives free from the constraint of medical rationality or the corruption of pharmaceutical agents. As modern individuals we are thoroughly and inescapably medical in our understanding of our bodies, our selves and our relationships with the world (Rose 2007). In *A Fine Line*, Dertadian records the capacity of contemporary consumers of medicine to develop their own forms of practical pharmacological expertise and actively negotiate a medicalized terrain in order to work toward their own goals. As he puts it, 'people's individualised appropriation of medical discourse and practice may well provide a compelling alternative to the psycho-pharmacological perspectives that have dominated much of the current literature about non-medical consumption.'

A Fine Line is a highly readable and engaging book based on up to date research and the author's extensive and detailed knowledge of the field. It introduces readers to the richness and complexity of an issue, which is too often discussed in simplistic and one-dimensional terms. Not only does it reveal the diverse forms of pharmaceutical self-intervention practiced by human beings in search of relief, self-improvement, pleasure and hope; it contributes to our understanding of the medical form of life that is inseparable from contemporary modes of existence.

Canberra, Australia

Associate Professor Helen Keane
Head of School, School of Sociology
Australian National University

References

Fox, N. J., & Ward, K. J. (2008). Pharma in the Bedroom... and the Kitchen.... The Pharmaceuticalisation of Daily Life. *Sociology of Health & Illness, 30*(6), 856–868.

Rose, N. (2007). Beyond Medicalisation. *Lancet, 369*(9562), 700–702.

Wing, S. (1994). Limits of Epidemiology. *Medicine and Global Survival, 1*(2), 74–86.

Preface

Are painkillers mundane medications safe for use to ameliorate human suffering? Or are they drugs of abuse that cause addiction and death? Do they ease pain, or do they cause it? The answer to these questions is a source of tension in professional and public understandings about the way people use painkillers.

It is hard to deny the benefit of the use of painkillers for chronic pain, in order to stem the constant, debilitating throb of pain that would otherwise not subside for physical health, nor for work or pleasure or rest. It is also hard to deny the pain these medications can *cause* to those who become dependent, and to the family and friends of those who lose their life to overdose. The later has, however, been brought into sharp focus by public health professionals ever since the slow-release opiate-based medication OxyContin® was released to market in 1996 in the US. The impact that the sale of this medication would have on American society and its public health would have been hard to fathom at the time.

Following the release of OxyContin®, Purdue Pharma, the company that owns the drug, utilized a sophisticated marketing machine that was largely directed by its majority owners, the Sackler family. A string of investigative journalism on the strategies used to market the drug has recently found that the company employed a series of deceptive and exploitative techniques to make it desirable to consumers and physicians alike. Those marketing deceptions proved incredibly successful for the Sackler family, with the medication going on to sell extremely well, making a fortune for Purdue Pharma.

Today, opiates are responsible for over 30,000 deaths per year in the US, with approximately half of those being caused by prescription medications. As a result, the marketing of OxyContin® and similar prescription opiates that have followed is regarded to be a commercial triumph that caused a public health tragedy.

While stories about the chronic pain patient, the dependent user and those who overdose present compelling accounts of painkillers as both the answer to and the cause of pain, they also represent the extremes of how these medications are consumed. This book will seek to shed light on more than these extremes by delving into the mundane ways in which painkillers are consumed in Australia, and seek to explain how they are connected to the way we understand and order our lives. It will foreground the historical and contemporary development of what has come to be known as the non-medical use of pharmaceuticals, and it will explore the everyday encounters with painkillers that make up people's lived experience of the use of these medications.

Through conceptual analysis and empirical investigation, this book illustrates how non-medical painkiller use is more contested and disparate than current public health research implies. While aspects of the archetypes of the desperate drug user who will 'use anything' or the 'naïve' user who runs into trouble with pain pills certainly feature, they are by no means the whole story. The work conducted in this book sits within critical drugs scholarship located at the intersection of cultural studies, sociology and criminology. These disciplines have explored the social construction, political economy and discursive formation of drug use. These approaches are used to explore tension between medical, neoliberal and consumer discourses about pain and pain medications, and are drawn out through reflections on research, media and public debate, as well as the lived experience of a mixed group of people living in Sydney who use painkillers non-medically, and were interviewed by the author.

The book is divided into two parts. The first focuses on official (historical, research, policy, etc.) discourses about non-medical consumption, while the second is largely concerned with the lived experience of those who use painkillers.

Part I of the book addresses key issues relevant to a robust critical analysis of non-medical painkiller use. This includes an assessment of relevant social theory, drug policy, research literature and conceptualizations of pain. Chapter 1 explores a range of concepts relevant to the field, including what a painkiller is, how the social sciences understand the medical profession, drug use and consumption more broadly, as well as the role of pleasure. Chapter 2 provides a historical account of the regulation of drugs in Australia by exploring key case studies about how approaches to drugs have changed over time, and especially as it relates to opiates and other analgesics. Chapter 3 provides a critical review of the available literature by assessing how it constructs the problem of non-medical 'abuse'. Chapter 4 canvases the way the definition of pain has been expanding in the medical, social and commercial domains.

Part II of the book involves analysis of qualitative interviews with people who use pain medications. These chapters trace how notions of individualized consumption inform medication use in a range of contexts, including intense work and recreational release, as well as the health practice of people who live in marginalized social conditions. Chapter 5 discusses young participants who use painkillers to 'chill out' as a way to respond to mild psychical discomfort, social unease and emotional discomfort. Chapter 6 addresses the way participants use pain medications as part of established cycles of production and consumption in contemporary society, in what is referred to as a 'work hard, play hard' dynamic. Chapter 7 discusses three case studies of participant's life histories that illustrate the complexities of chronic pain and its entanglement with different types of dependence. Chapter 8 explores the lives of two participants who no longer use drug as a way to examine the limitations of addiction as the primary concept used to understand opiate consumption in general and non-medical painkiller use in particular.

Penrith, Australia George C. Dertadian

Acknowledgements

I am endlessly grateful to the participants who volunteered their life experiences to this project. Thank you for sharing your stories and trusting me with them. Your candor has made this book what it is.

Many thanks and much love to my ever supportive family and friends. To my dearest Gariné, your love makes life easy and I'm so glad I wrote this with you by my side.

I would like to acknowledge the support and funding provided by the Institute for Culture and Society, Western Sydney University (WSU) during my Ph.D., which comprises the research on which this book is based. I would also like to thank the School of Social Sciences and Psychology, WSU, for providing a stable and supportive professional environment in which to develop the ideas in the Doctorate into the form they now take in this book.

Special thanks are owed to Stephen Tomsen for encouraging me to write the book; for his personal and professional support, both during his time as my Ph.D. supervisor and since.

I also would like to express my gratitude to Lisa Maher for giving me the opportunity to continue to research this topic after graduating from the Doctorate and acknowledge the contribution my time working with you has made to the ideas explored in this book.

Warm thanks are also owed to Helen Keane for not only agreeing to write the forward to this book, but also for being such a prominent intellectual inspiration on the content of the book.

I am greatful to the wonderful members of our qualitative reading group, Kari, Kenneth, Jake and Alison, for their intellectual inspiration and cherished friendship.

Lastly, I would like to thank the supportive community of Australian critical drugs scholars, on whose shoulders I stood when writing this book.

Contents

Abbreviations

ABS	Australian Bureau of Statistics
ADHD	Attention Deficit Hyperactivity Disorder
AIC	Australian Institute of Criminology
APA	American Psychiatric Association
APC	Aspirin, Phenacetin and Caffeine Products
ASMI	Australian Self Medication Industry
AVIL	Australian Injecting and Illicit Drug Users League
DEA	Drug Enforcement Agency (US)
DORA	Drugs and Poisons Information System, Online Reporting Software
DSM	Diagnostic and Statistical Manual for Mental Disorders
DUMA	Drug Use Monitoring in Australia
ERRCD	Electronic Recording and Reporting of Controlled Drugs
IASP	International Association for the Study of Pain
IDRS	Illicit Drug Reporting System
INCB	International Narcotics Control Board
MSIC	Medically Supervised Injecting Centre
NDARC	National Drug and Alcohol Research Centre (Australia)
NDS	National Drug Strategy (Australia)
NDSHS	National Drugs Strategy Household Survey (Australia)
NIDA	National Institute on Drug Abuse (USA)

NSP	Needle and Syringe Program(s)
OST	Opioid substitution treatment
PBAC	Pharmaceutical Benefits Advisory Committee
PBS	Pharmaceutical Benefits Scheme
SAMHSA	Substance Abuse and Mental Health Services Administration (US)
SUD	Substance Use Disorder
TGA	Therapeutic Goods Administration

Drugs Glossary

Regulatory Status	Chemical name	Brand name	Colloquial terms
Prohibited substance	Cannabis		Dope
	Dexamphetamine sulfate		Dexamphetamine
	Diamorphine		Heroin; Gear; Junk
	Methylenedioxy methamphetamine		MDMA; Ecstasy; e
	Psilocybin mushrooms		Magic mushrooms
Prescription required	Alprazolam	Xanax	
	Methadone		Done
	Morphine	MS-Contin	
	Oxycodone	Endone; OxyContin; OxyNorm	Oxy; Hillbilly heroin
	Paracetamol; Codeine phosphate	Panadeine Forte; Tramadol	
	Paracetamol; Ccodeine phosphate hemihydrate; Doxylamine succinate	Mersyndol; Mersyndol Forte	
	Quetiapine	Seroquel	
	Temazepam	Restoril; Normison; Nortem	
Available without prescription*	Paracetamol	Panadol	
	Paracetamol; Codeine phosphate	Nurofen; Nurofen Plus; Panadeine Extra	

*This glossary is a guide for the prescription status of the medications listed at the time of interview.

Part I

The Way We Think About Non-Medical Use

1

Introduction: Understanding Painkiller Use in Contemporary Society

Painkillers were not always seen as dangerous drugs. Less than 20 years ago, these medications were largely regarded to be innocuous pharmaceuticals safely prescribed by the doctor. Since the early 2000s however, growing concern about the ability for painkillers to be 'abused' emerged alongside reports of spates of 'illicit' pharmaceutical opiate consumption and related harm in Missouri (Harris et al. 2002), rural Kentucky (Tunnell 2005) and California, among other areas (Whelan et al. 2011). Since the early 2010s, concern about the harms of painkiller consumption has only escalated, with the non-medical use of pharmaceutical opiates being referred to as the 'opiate crisis' and as a 'deadly drug epidemic'. What has made this starker to health practitioners is the fact that opiate overdose trends in the US have seen the largest increases in deaths among populations that have traditionally low rates of drug use; this includes Caucasians, the middle-aged, those in the middle class and women (Rudd et al. 2016; Bohnert et al. 2011). The US context has seen increases in emergency room presentations related to opiate overdose (Yokell et al. 2014) and opiate dependence (Carise et al. 2007). Research also indicates that many of the country's youngest generation of heroin users were first introduced to opiates through pharmaceuticals (Carlson et al. 2016; McCabe et al. 2007). Comparable patterns of

G. C. Dertadian, *A Fine Line*,
https://doi.org/10.1007/978-981-13-1975-4_1

harm have also emerged in epidemiological data from other parts of the world (Fischer et al. 2010).

The tragic circumstances that surround the harm being caused by opiate consumption in the US have also made its way into the popular imagination, with use of colloquial terms like 'hillbilly heroin', 'rich man's heroin' or simply 'killer', reimagining medications such as OxyContin® in the image of the urban 'junkie' that has haunted North American drug research for decades (Acker 2002). It has also inspired a succession of documentary films (Coker and Mackson 2017; Carney 2010) and autobiographical books (Lyon 2009; Stein 2009) devoted to telling the story of 'normal' people who use this 'dangerous drug' and have become 'addicts'. Pop culture accounts of opiate use and abuse have focused in particular on the way the recent painkiller crisis has changed the image of what an 'addict' is, often noting with surprise that 'anyone can become addicted to painkillers'.

While many have declared opiate-related harm in the US an 'epidemic' (Conrad et al. 2015; Jones et al. 2015), public health data do not support the notion that the same conditions of harm have emerged in Australia. While Australia has seen significant increases in the prescription of pharmaceutical opiates (Blanch et al. 2014), opiate overdose deaths remained relatively low for some time (Roxburgh et al. 2011). Data from a variety of national monitoring programs also indicate that pharmaceutical opiate-related overdose deaths remain relatively low in Australia when compared to heroin (Roxburgh et al. 2011). Moreover, Australian research suggests that non-medical pharmaceutical opiate users tend to be people with an established history of injection drug use prior to first injecting pharmaceuticals (Nielsen et al. 2015; Degenhardt et al. 2006). Yet rates of heroin use in Australia have remained low (Coghlan et al. 2015), meaning that there is little evidence to suggest that pharmaceutical opiate use is seeding heroin use in the way that it has found to be in the US. However, since 2008 there has been a noticeable increase in overdose deaths related to pharmaceutical opiates, largely driven by increases in Fentanyl overdoses (Roxburgh et al. 2017).

Differences between the Australian and US context are illustrative of the fact that many questions remain unanswered by the public health information available about death and dependence. While epidemiology tells us that pharmaceutical opiate consumption represents a serious public health crisis in the US and an emerging problem in Australia, it cannot tell us why: What are the differences in the profiles of harm between the US and Australian contexts? Why do people use these medications in the first place? Answering these questions requires a different approach than traditional public health's inclination to record rates of morbidity and mortality can provide: it requires paying attention to the history of drug policy and research; it requires an awareness of the structures that shape the society in which painkillers are consumed; and it requires a genuine engagement with the stories of people who actually use these medications.

This chapter begins the task of this book by outlining the conceptual tools needed to analyze non-medical consumption of pain medications beyond the headlines about addiction and overdose. These tools will be used to articulate how the use of painkillers illustrates a fine line between medical and illegal use, pain relief and pleasurable consumption. This chapter will thus set out the theoretical background on which the book is based and the social conditions on which it comments. It will explore the social construction of the term 'painkiller', provide a summary of relevant theory related to the analysis of medicine, drug use and consumption in late-modern societies, as well as articulate the way pleasure will be dealt with throughout the book and how the research was conducted.

What Is a Painkiller?

In simple terms, 'painkiller' refers to a variable range of pharmaceuticals that are prescribed or used for the relief of pain. However, it is important to recognize that the categorization of a drug as a painkiller is highly context dependent, since it often includes controlled substances that are illicit unless prescribed. This necessarily positions medical practitioners and authorities as the crucial mediating agency in access to pain relief. The construction of a drug as a painkiller is therefore a social and legal process that is frequently elided in medical and scientific accounts.

The medical literature describes painkillers as a group of drugs that act on the peripheral and central nervous systems to achieve analgesia—relief from pain. This drug type is also commonly referred to as analgesic medication. Most analgesic medications are at least partial synthetic formulations derived but not directly extracted from the opium poppy. Analgesic medications available in Australia include paracetamol, ibuprofen and, the most popular, opioids (or opiates). Morphine is the major psychoactive chemical in opiate-based substances and is found in both its prescription (oxycodone, hydromorphone, etc.) and over-the-counter (codeine) variations. The chemical structure of opiates are not, however, limited to analgesic medications. The illicit drug heroin is also considered an opiate because it shares a similar chemical structure to many prescription analgesics and produces similar mechanisms of action (Robson 2009).

Medical accounts of pain relief draw heavily from scientific classifications based on the drug's chemical structure or effect on the body. The typical scientific taxonomy of drugs based on chemical structure will include the following categories: opioids (or opiates), sedatives, stimulants, cannabinoids, hallucinogens and volatile inhalants. The opiate is the most common drug type used for the relief of pain, although sedatives have a long history in pain relief (Hughes 2008: 37). Cannabinoids have also been presented as having pain-relieving potential, particularly in the case of chronic pain or recovery from cancer (Iversen and Chapman 2002; Holdcroft et al. 1997). It is, however, important to recognize that not all drugs fall clearly into one category, nor do all drugs in one category produce the same mechanisms of action. For instance, alcohol produces both sedative and stimulant effects on the body (Hendler et al. 2013). Moreover, knowledge about the physiology of the human body is limited in ways that make it difficult to account for a drug's impact on multiple parts of the brain (Degrandpre and White 1996).

Given such limitations, classification systems often end up relying on "social categories like legality, therapeutic potential and potential for abuse" (Keane 2002). Consequently, classificatory structures can ignore the chemical and functional similarities of some drugs in favor of their social construction. Social constructions like legality and therapeutic potential are the main way in which painkillers are categorized, both in lay and in professional contexts. One of the implications of this is that symbolic distance is often placed between licit and illicit forms of the same drug type.

The distinction made between pharmaceutical analgesic and illicit drugs also involves elements of the regulatory systems that control the international supply of opiates and other drugs. From a succession of international treaties during (and before) the 1960s, the International Narcotics Control Board (INCB) classified different drug formulations into a system of categories called schedules. Each schedule requires different levels of reporting to the INCB. The schedule system structures the availability of the substances classified as opiates and their use for the treatment of pain. Domestic legislation provides its own system of schedules for the medical and indeed criminal regulation of opiates, which have both licit and illicit uses according to law. These regulatory and legislative structures borrow from and reproduce medical discourses that construct certain drugs as therapeutic. However, international law does not determine domestic criminal law or medical conduct. Instead, policies within nation-states are partly structured around international regulation and an increasingly globalized medical profession.

The subjective experience about what may constitute relief from pain also considerably expands the colloquial scope of the term painkiller. For example, the 'painkilling' effects of alcohol are recognized in culturally entrenched forms of drinking to 'kill the pain' or 'numb the pain', although alcohol is not medically prescribed for pain relief. A substance's status as 'medication' is therefore intricately tied to its role in a medical narrative of treatment.

A painkiller can be defined in different ways in different contexts. Analgesic medications are understood as therapeutic technologies because they are distinguished from their more stigmatized (opiate) counterparts. A complex combination of legislative structures, professional practice and even commercial interests (Blackett and Robins 2001; Fisher 2003) frame the way particular substances are either used in medical treatment or ascribed a criminal classification. The 'painkiller' is best understood as a particular enactment of legislative, pharmacological and discursive frameworks surrounding medical practice.

The way painkillers are consumed, and how this is structured by the conditions of contemporary society are a key concern of this book. The sections that follow will explore how the conditions of late-modernity shape medical discourse and consumption practices.

Medicine and Medicalization

In order to understand the way pain is defined, it is important to examine scholarship on the medical profession and the way it understands health, the body and the human condition. This section will explore foundational aspects of and recent developments in social science scholarship on medicine, in order to contextualize key ideas that will be drawn on throughout Part I of the book.

Since the 1950s, sociological research has been interested in the influence of the medical profession within society. One of the key features of this interest in medicine, and the medical profession has been the notion of 'medicalization'. The term medicalization refers to the process by which human problems become defined and treated as medical conditions (Conrad 2008). The medicalization thesis was originally developed during the 1950s and 1960s in response to the rapid growth of the medical profession at the time (Lupton 1997). Social researchers began to notice that the medical perspective was encroaching on a range of 'deviant' social behaviors, which were increasingly the subject of medical intervention. Much of its earliest uses in sociology developed Marxist (Illich 1976) and feminist critiques (Ehrenreich and English 1973, 1978) of the way the medical profession acted as an agent of social control.

During this time, psychiatry in particular was accused of pathologizing drug consumption as a 'female problem' (Cooperstock 1976). Higher rates of women seeking physician services, as well as being prescribed and using more medication, led feminist scholars to the conclusion that conceptualizations of 'drug taking behaviour be based on a broader perspective than that of purely individual considerations' (Cooperstock 1978). Women's experiences of oppression were either ignored (prompting some women to 'self-medicate') or individualized as symptoms of ill-health/emotional instability. Feminist accounts of medicalization thus linked women's use of substances, both licit and illicit, to the widespread pathologization of women and their bodies.

At the same time, analysis of the pathologization of mental states became an influential strand of critical medicalization scholarship, with a disparate group of scholars forming, what came to be known as the antipsychiatry movement. The work of influential thinkers such as Szasz (1961, 1970) and Foucault (1973, 1988) is regarded as important precursors to the antipsychiatry movement (Dain 1989). Antipsychiatry focused on the social control elements of the psychiatric profession and argued that medical discourse was being used to disguise moral judgments about the behavior being 'treated' (Pearson 1975). During the 1980s, American sociologist Conrad and Schneider (1980) outlined how a range of 'deviant' behaviors, including alcohol and opiate consumption, were becoming the subject of medical intervention. At the same time, Crawford observed a heightened ideological concern about health in industrial societies, describing how an age of 'healthism' was informing the medicalization of everyday life.

Since the introduction of medicalization as an analytical tool social science, researchers have indicated a need to diversify the concept in response to changing circumstances. Notable attempts to capture nuanced elements of medicalization include the technological focus of 'biomedicalization' (Clarke et al. 2003), 'geneticization' in the construction of mental illness (Phelan 2005) and the importance of market mechanisms highlighted with 'pharmaceuticalization' (Bell and Figert 2012). The concept of pharmaceuticalization will be particularly relevant to the analysis in this book.

One of the central arguments surrounding a shift toward a pharmaceuticalization framework is the significance of industry entanglement with modern health care. Much controversy has, for instance, surrounded the relationship between the pharmaceutical industry and prescribing physicians (Wazana 2000). US studies have indicated that "interactions with the industry were found to start as early as medical school and to continue well into practice" (Wazana 2000: 375). In 2004, Conrad and Leiter argue that:

> Until the last decade or so, sociologists rarely examined medicine as any kind of marketplace. But it is becoming clear that, with the development of managed care, corporatized medicine, and the rise of the biotechnology industry, medical markets are increasingly important in the analysis of health care. (2004: 160)

Though the regulation of 'medical markets' remains ultimately with the medical profession, thus operating outside the conditions of traditional 'free markets', recent shifts have seen consumer demand play a leading role (Conrad and Leiter 2004; Williams et al. 2008).

However, the medical profession, and increasingly the pharmaceutical industry also assume a determining role in what is considered a medical problem appropriate for pharmaceutical intervention. There are professional and commercial interests involved in what is given medical attention and what medications are made available for treatment. Thus, the way medical knowledge formulates health and illness is not a self-evident elaboration of the human condition. The conditions of modern society produce a range of effects on the human subject that are only selectively ascribed a medical label. Medicalization scholarship provides important tools to contextualize the social constructions and political economies that inform our culture's approach to pain and the consumption of pharmaceuticals. Aspects of medicalization scholarship will be drawn on throughout Part I of the book to explore the way medical definitions of pain have been expanding to encompass difficult and uncertain social conditions.

Critical Drugs Scholarship

Social research perspectives also have a long history of exploring the relationship between medical discourse and drug consumption. Social science research in sociology and criminology has informed the empirical assessment of drug use and the development of contemporary critical drugs scholarship. This section will outline a set of key literature that provides the conceptual tools for analysis of policy and research on drug use.

The social construction of drug use is an important element of critical drugs scholarship. Research about social deviance became foundational to the lasting tradition of the University of Birmingham's Centre for Contemporary Cultural Studies (CCCS) (Cohen 1972; Hebdige 1979), as well as the critical criminology movement (Cohen and Young 1973; Taylor et al. 1973). It is within these traditions that critical scholarship has developed skepticism of the notion of opiates (and other drugs) as 'drugs of abuse'. This is not to deny that people may experience problems with drugs, but to seek to situate that experience within its social and cultural context. This includes the labeling and stigmatization of people who use drugs within political, media and medical discourse.

The critical tradition of drug research can be traced to Young's *The Drug Takers* (1971), which argued that the practices of people who use drugs formed a system of 'subterranean' values that closely resemble the conventional value systems of 'late' and 'post'-industrial societies. Young observes that the British citizenry 'must produce in order to consume, and consume in order to produce. The interrelationship between formal and subterranean values is therefore seen in a new light: hedonism, for instance, is closely tied to productivity' (1971: 128). Such an account demonstrates how kinds of drug use are constructed to be hedonistic because of their relationship with socially desirable notions of productivity. The social construction of drug use is thus necessary to consider when discussing how kinds of pharmaceutical consumption are constructed to be medical and others non-medical.

By the 1980s, the social construction of drug use had become an established area of study. Rather than continuing to reiterate the social construction of drug use, researchers began to focus on the elements of that construction. Taking their lead from Zinberg's influential study with heroin users, *Drug, Set, and Setting* (1986), qualitative drugs research began to focus on the 'social context' of drug use (Rhodes and Moore 2001). Zinberg's work provided one of the first, and certainly the most influential theoretical frameworks of drug consumption that incorporated considerations of the pharmacological, psychological and social (Moore 1993). Drug researchers began to emphasize how diverse contexts produce particular forms of drug taking. For instance, research turned its attention to the lives of sex workers in a street-based drug market in Brooklyn (Maher 1997), and to street-level crack dealers in the 'ghetto' neighborhood of East Harlem (Bourgois 1995). These kinds of political economies of drug consumption describe how the construction of particular forms of drug use is embedded in certain social contexts.

Poststructuralist contributions from cultural studies (and related disciplines) have built on the social and political accounts of drug use discussed thus far by highlighting the role of discourse. Poststructuralist accounts help to explain how social constructions and political economies can be molded and transformed by the discourses used to articulate them (Race 2009; Sulkunen 2002). Following from the notion that a drug's effects are contextually contingent, poststructuralist drug scholarship has made important contributions to critical perspectives on addiction, in particular maintaining skepticism over the notion that addiction is a single knowable entity that medicine can simply discover and treat (Alexander and Roberts 2012). Poststructuralism tells us that addiction is a historically and culturally contingent phenomenon that is the product of a diverse set of social, political and discursive formations (Redfield and Brodie 2002).

Keane's *What's Wrong with Addiction?* (2002) is a particularly significant work in the field that problematizes cultural formulations of drug dependence as 'addiction'. Keane's work identifies the various conceptualizations of 'drug addiction' found in, for instance, scientific classifications of drugs, pain medicine literature (Keane and Hamill 2010), psychiatric diagnostic practice (Fraser et al. 2014), and the self-help and 12-step philosophies (Keane 2002). The discursive element is most clearly demonstrated in her exploration of the expansion of addiction discourse to forms of 'strong attachments, powerful urges, preoccupation and social harm' (Keane 2002: 63) that are in no way limited to drug use—what has been termed behavioral addictions. Referring to the emergence of food and sex 'addictions' in psychiatric and popular discourse, Keane asks:

> Can food and sex act like psychoactive drugs and alter people's psychological and physiological functioning? Or are these addictions simply moral

> judgements about 'bad' ways of eating and having sex dressed up in the language of disease? If addiction is not determined by a particular property of the object of addiction, as the recent proliferation of addictions suggests, does this mean that everything is potentially addictive? (Keane 2002: 5)

Of course Keane's goal is not to determine whether 'addiction' is *really* a property of the drug or a generalizable category of disease. Instead, her work acknowledges that 'our tools for making knowledge help to constitute the very phenomena under observation' (Keane et al. 2011: 875).

In the tradition of such critical drugs scholarship, this study will unpack the assumptions behind 'official' understandings (Burton and Carlen 2013) of non-medical consumption as a 'social problem' (Bacchi 2009). It examines the institutional authority and expert purchase of official discourses of medical and political knowledge about drug consumption. This approach draws from poststructuralist traditions of discourse analysis that critique the way the subject of policy and research is presented as fixed or preexisting (Barker and Galasinski 2001). The analysis conducted does not simply treat expert perspectives and policy accounts as a mode of addressing drug use. Instead, it explores how the discourses that make up 'official' understandings of non-medical consumption partly shape the phenomena being articulated.

Consumption in the 'Age of Anxiety'

Consumption is an important part of postindustrial societies. People are encouraged by a wide variety of sources to purchase and enjoy a range of commodities (Ritzer 2001, 2005). Advertisements from large companies are splashed over the cityscape of urban spaces and are increasingly embedded in online formats. Encouragement to consume is everywhere. There are, however, limits to consumption, and in the contemporary context 'proper' consumption is most often viewed under a framework of rational-medical discourse. The influence of the medical perspective in this respect is linked to enlightenment thinking about rationality and moderation (Reith 2004). The structural components of modernity, including though not exclusively the influence of the medical perspective, thus frame the way people consume. This section will explore the frameworks used to analyze consumption in contemporary society that are drawn on throughout the book.

Since the foundational work of Karl Marx (1848) established a critique of the exploitation of the labor (and production) of the working class, social theorists have noted a shift toward the role of consumption in the enduring influence of the capitalist economic system (Ritzer 2014; Horkheimer et al. 1944). Another key feature of modernist traditions is enlightenment thinking and the prominence it places on the liberal subject—who must have equal and full access to free choice in their lives in order to be able to express and be themselves (Kelly 2005). Under the liberal philosophy, social conditions that impede choice are seen to compromise the autonomy of the individual and are largely regarded as oppressive. In much liberal philosophy, there is thus a strong emphasis on the role of the state in ensuring the conditions of society allow for freedom of choice. The ideal of the freedom to consume is thus also central to the formation of the liberal subject in modern capitalist societies. There is, however, a range of limitations to the liberal philosophy that should be noted. Liberalism assumes that its subject is a rational agent whose choices, given the appropriate social condition, can be made independent of the social context in which they occur. The idea that everyone in our culture has equal access to all forms of information, especially about health, is, however, hotly contested (Benoit et al. 2010).

Liberalism is also an evolving tradition in Western thought. Over the past thirty years, the concept of neoliberalism has emerged as a prominent element of economic and social policy in many late capitalist societies. Like classical liberalism, neoliberalism espouses the ideals of freedom of choice. However, for neoliberalism the freedom of the individual is the responsibility of the individual. In the context of health, neoliberalism demands a radically individualized subject that shifts the responsibility for well-being away from social conditions and onto the individual (Petersen and Lupton 1996). People are instructed to make 'healthy life choices' by being an 'informed consumer' of health products (Petersen et al. 2010). Unlike classical liberalism, the neoliberal philosophy has tended to devolve the responsibility of the state for health and social welfare by placing the onus on the individual.

The development of neoliberal thought has emerged alongside other transformations in the modern condition observed by social theorists toward the end of the twentieth century. Contemporary theorists have emphasized a fracturing of the way people relate to modernist institutions. Beck (1992) argues that capitalist and medical institutions are less reliable as foundations of community and identity. For instance, the workforce is increasingly casualized in late capitalist economies (Bauman 2007) and medical authority is encouraged to be verified by 'doing your research' and 'getting a second opinion' (Germov 2009). For Beck, and those who followed in a similar tradition such as Beck et al. (1994), what is referred to as risk societies are thought to be constantly concerned with potential future risk and thus operate in a mode of uncertainty. The terms 'post' (Baudrillard 1998), 'high' (Giddens 1991) and 'reflexive' (Beck 1992) modernity have also been used to describe similar transformations in the modern condition as:

> an era that is characterized by restructuring of economic and labour market processes and the diversification and fragmentation of social, familial, and community relations. It is dominated by increased insecurity, flux, and risk in social life. (Reith 2004: 230)

The fragmentation of the traditional structures of modernity is also thought to be implicated in increasingly individualized responses to problems that can largely be understood as socially produced (Bauman 2001). This is particularly conducive to processes of responsibilization endorsed by neoliberal discourse.

The way in which modern societies encourage constant evaluation of possible risks illustrates the way the modern condition is implicated in notions of anxiousness. Salecl has more recently observed how contemporary capitalism relies on the anxieties of the consumer (2004: 30), noting that, within late capitalist economies cycles of consumption rely on anxiety about 'proper' feminine appearance or middle-class ideals of 'healthy living'. Following observations about risk and increasing uncertainty in late-modern societies, Bauman has formulated a thesis about a shift from 'solid' to a 'liquid' stage of modernity (2003, 2006, 2007). Bauman describes 'liquid modern' as a "society in which the conditions under which its members act change faster than it takes the ways of acting to consolidate into habits and routines" (2013: 1). In liquid modern societies, the individual is placed in a process of unending demand for flexibility to negotiate constant change: 'In such a society, the sentiments of existential insecurity and scattered fears of diffuse dangers are, inevitably, endemic' (Bauman 2007: 57).

Foucault's work on governmentality in the 1970s has also been used to trace changes in modernity and its impact on issues of governance. Governmentality scholarship has broadly traced how 'modern states [have] moved from rule by crude force to sophisticated governance based on (shaped) consent' (Ferlie et al. 2012). This work has made significant contributions to the characterization of the late-modern era as a period of fragmented identity politics and individualized self-discipline. Governmentality scholars have applied the concept to contemporary approaches to health. Observations about a trend toward neoliberalism in late-modern societies have prompted analysis about the state's retreat from health care, focusing instead on individual responsibility for health (Lupton 2014; Woolhouse et al. 2012). Governmentality scholarship has subsequently become influential in the analysis of the neoliberal governance of disease transmission (Fraser and Seear 2013), overdose prevention (Moore 2004) and supervised injecting sites (Fischer et al. 2004), among a range of non-drug-related health practices (Petersen et al. 2010).

The constantly adaptable subject demanded by the social conditions described in this section is part of, what Bauman refers to as the 'age of anxiety'—a time in which consumption is presented as a way to ease constant worry about fleeting identities and unstable social arrangements. In this way, this book refers to anxiety not in its pathological sense, but as an expected human response to uncertainty. The theoretical accounts discussed here provide a framework for analyzing how consumption is used in this age of anxiety to negotiate the constant demand for flexibility in the pursuit of ideal health and productive consumption.

In Pursuit of Pleasure

Part of the goal of this book is to articulate the way painkillers are used in the pursuit of pleasure. In order to do so, it is useful to first canvass drug use literature about pleasure. At the outset, it is important to note that discussion of pleasure is underrepresented in research about drug use (Holt and Treloar 2008). Pleasure is curiously excluded from discussion of the nature of addiction (Keane 2002; Campbell 2007), policy and governance related to drug consumption (Moore 2008; O'Malley and Valverde 2004), as well as the analysis of user accounts (Moore and Valverde 2010; Hunt et al. 2007). A common explanation for sidestepping pleasure in accounts of drug use is the way it is presented as "ameliorating pain rather than causing pleasure" (Fraser 2008: 410–411).

The notion that problematic drug use in particular is about numbing pain instead of producing pleasure is used in the individualized accounts of psychoanalysis and the structural explanations of social science. Psychological explanations about drug use tend to argue that drugs are used not for the euphoric physical effect they have on the person consuming them, but as a way to 'self-medicate' the pain of personal trauma and mental illness (Hall and Queener 2007; Markoua et al. 1998; Khantzian 1997). Avoiding the contentiousness of pleasure in favor of medicalized discourses about trauma and illness allows for an account of drug use and addiction that is more politically expedient—in other words, policymakers are more likely to procure resources to help people who use drugs if those people are presented as vulnerable and damaged (White 1998). While much of this work is certainly well intentioned, conflating trauma and drug use can reduce problematic drug use to evidence of trauma (Fraser 2008). Much qualitative research has demonstrated that this is an oversimplification of motivations for drug consumption (Jarvinen and Ravn 2011).

Social scientists on the other hand have argued that structural factors such as race and class determine problematic drug use because it is a response to the suffering of social marginalization. While there is plenty of evidence to suggest that structural factors that marginalize people who use drugs have an impact on levels of harm (Rhodes 2009; Rhodes et al. 2005), this approach can conflate drug use and other 'social problems' such as crime and delinquency in ways that are not accurate nor useful (Seddon 2006; Beckett 1994). Applying this kind of deterministic approach can also leave the impression that people who use drugs and the problems they experience are 'exceptional' or unique, rather than understanding them to be part of the broader political economy in which the harms they experience are embedded.

Lastly, a broader critique of this way of understanding drug use (as lacking pleasure but providing analgesia) is that it reduces the agentive capacity of people who use drugs. If drug use is only ever a response to mental anguish or social marginalization, then qualitative evidence about the capacity for self-directed choices about health and pleasure are left out of the equitation (Moore and Fraser 2006). These positions have sought to defuse the social unease with and political objection to the notion that people enjoy the drugs they consume by saying that pain relief and pleasure are incompatible phenomena. Through an assessment of the literature on pain and suffering, and an analysis of interview material with people who use painkillers non-medically, this book will instead argue that relief from pain and experiences of pleasure are not mutually exclusive.

Criminological research has also provided broader explanations for the pursuit of pleasure through drug consumption. In acknowledging the fragmentation of modern life discussed in the previous section, social theorists have explored the notion that forms of pleasurable drug use can be conceived of as a response to the conditions of late-modernity. In an influential 1990 article in the American Journal of Sociology, Lyng formulated the theory of edgework, which posits that some people derive pleasure from physical activities that involve uncertainty and risk taking. Much of the early edgework literature focused on the way practices like extreme sports (Jonas 1999) and illicit drug use (Collison 1996) are forms of resistance to the fragmented and uncertain circumstances of the conditions of modernity. Edgework scholars argue that these 'risk takers' re-appropriate the detrimental elements of uncertainty to 'take control' of risk, that they subvert the detriments of risk by deriving pleasure from it (Holyfield and Fine 1997; Ferrell and Stewart-Huidobro 1996). While this approach forms a significant part of edgework scholarship, an opposing, though not entirely irreconcilable tradition has also emerged to suggest that edgework is less an escape from, but rather an extension of the conditions of late-modernity (Lyng 2004). Pointing to the centrality of the individual in negotiating the risks of modern life, scholars have suggested that the pleasurable 'edgework' of drug use may be permissively encouraged by late-modern society. Edgework scholarship is primarily based on qualitative research about the lived experience of people who engage in pleasurable risk taking.

While pleasure is scarcely discussed in drug research, people who use drugs regularly cite it as an important reason for ongoing consumption. Alfred Lindesmith (1938), who has been dubbed the 'father of the sociology of addiction', was the first twentieth-century researcher to refer to, what he termed the 'pleasure user' or the 'joy popper'. Though not extensively discussed in his work, the 'pleasure user' was specifically distinguished as someone who used heroin for pleasure only occasionally, and was not dependent on the drug. Howard Becker's classic book *Outsiders* (1963) goes further, arguing that the drug itself is not enough to produce the pleasures of cannabis—instead arguing that people who smoke the drug must engage in a learning process, through social interaction, before they can actually become 'high' and thus experience the drug's pleasures. This has been extended on in Zinberg's (1986) influential account of 'controlled intoxicant use' and subsequent accounts of 'functional users' (Lende et al. 2007; Degenhardt et al. 2005). These social constructionist accounts present the pleasure of drug use as an inherent part of the drug being consumed and describe social processes by which users learn or discover the pleasure of drugs in 'functional' ways.

Beyond social constructionism, poststructuralist accounts have also explored the idea that the pleasures of drug use are not inherent in the drug, instead arguing that pleasure is a phenomenon that emerges through relationships between drugs, people and their environments. Small bodies of contemporary research have explored the performative and corporeal elements of the pleasures of drug use. Research about raves, dance parties and nighttime entertainment has illustrated that these are spaces of transgression, where young people derive pleasure from feeling and becoming 'different' to how they are in everyday life

(Winlow and Hall 2006). In these contexts, a range of social practices such as 'dancing and interacting with strangers… were reportedly facilitated with the use of different drugs' (Duff 2008: 386). A key element of these accounts of pleasure is that the practices that surround drug use are themselves pleasurable. Pleasure is enacted through the dancing and extroverted socializing that drug use facilitates in rave and club cultures (Hunt et al. 2007). Thus, it is worth noting that the pleasure of one's experience on drugs is also about the practices that drug use makes possible or easier to access.

Scholarship on the pleasures of medication consumption tends to support poststructuralist accounts of drug pleasures. Race's (2009) seminal work in this area has theorized how public health discourse about drug consumption has become a site upon which the neoliberal State can police the apparent excesses of the amoral market. In his work, illicit drug use is symbolic of the moral ills of unbridled consumption that is used to guise the harms of unrestricted commercial consumption. Race also finds that pragmatic citizens of the neoliberal State thus find no need to regard health as antithetical to pleasure. This is articulated by the consumption practices of a group of gay men who use drugs to foster the pleasures of social interaction and sexual encounters, as well as engage in preventative health measures. In another qualitative study about young people's initiation into non-medical pharmaceutical use, Bundy and Quintero discuss how pleasure is rarely experienced at first use. The study found that a common experience among participants was that pleasure emerged out of regular and informed use, rather than from the pharmaceutical qualities of the drug itself. The authors note that pharmaceuticals had 'durable effects [that] emerged as practiced users begin to parse the pharmaceutical experience' (Bundy and Quintero 2017: 112). This meant that when using medications, the way study participants "constitute these experiences as desirable or satisfying comes to have a wide range of meanings beyond simply 'getting high'" (Bundy and Quintero 2017: 109).

Through an assessment of the way participants use painkillers in various ways to pursue pleasure, this book will argue that relief from pain is not always so different from experiences of pleasure. It explores the way people who use painkillers pursue pleasure, whether by indulging in inebriate consumption of analgesic medications or by using them to alter or prolong other kinds of pleasurable activities. This means that, rather than simply focusing on notions of hedonistic pleasure, in the context of this book 'pleasure' may also refer to relief from feelings of uncertainty and insecurity as much as it does to the euphoria of an opiate high. These are not of course mutually exclusive conceptualizations of pleasure, and as we shall see throughout the book, people who use opiates and other pain medications often experience a complex mixture of pleasurable feelings related variously to social ease, temporary emotional numbing and enjoyable inebriation.

Research Approach

The study conducted in this book includes two parts. Part I involves the analysis of historical, research and documentary material, which is used to inform the interpretation of interview data in Part II. Part I unpacks the assumptions behind 'official' understandings (Burton and Carlen 2013) of non-medical consumption as a 'social problem' (Bacchi 2009). It examines the institutional authority and expert purchase of 'official discourses' of medical and political knowledge about drug consumption. This approach draws from poststructuralist traditions of discourse analysis that critique the way the subject of policy and research is presented as fixed or preexisting (Barker and Galasinski 2001). The analysis conducted does not regard expert perspectives and policy accounts as a mode of addressing drug use. Instead, it explores how the discourses that make up 'official' understandings of non-medical consumption partly shape the phenomena being articulated.

Part I also involves critical analysis of a variety of fields of expert knowledge. Key documents influential across policy and research are targeted because of the role they play in defining non-medical use. For instance, the American Psychiatric Association's (APA) Diagnostic and Statistical Manual for Mental Disorders (DSM) is analyzed for its impact on discourses of anxiety and substance dependence. Policy documents and material from key institutions are also explored. The work of the US-based National Institute on Drug Abuse (NIDA), as well as

Australian institutions such as the National Drug and Alcohol Research Centre (NDARC) and the Australian Institute of Criminology (AIC), are surveyed for their contribution to, and construction of, debates about non-medical use and addiction.

This analysis is carried out through close reading (Bowen 2009) and analysis of key archival material, policy documents and research literature (Silverman 2013). Broad developments in the approach to and meaning of opiate and other drug consumption are surveyed in a range of relevant material (Saukko 2003). Shifts in the significance of drug use and medical authority over pharmaceutical consumption are drawn out through analysis of media, policy and political documentation. Research on the social and legal development of drug policy and social welfare is used to inform the interpretation of historical documentation.

The empirical material in Part II of the book draws on a project that involved talking to people who engage in non-medical consumption, in the form of qualitative semi-structured interviews. Interviews sought to answer key questions, such as: Who consumes painkillers non-medically?; How do they think and talk about what they are doing? Participants were sourced from health care facilities ($n = 2$), tertiary education institutions ($n = 2$), the internet ($n = 17$) and personal approaches ($n = 4$). This took the form of flyers that were also adapted to the format of three websites: airtasker.com, facebook.com and gumtree.com. The project targeted a variety of people who use painkillers that ranged from occasional, to regular/recreational and dependent. Twenty-seven interviews were conducted with 25 participants (2 participants were interviewed twice).

User narratives were gathered through semi-structured qualitative interviews, organized around guiding questions about life history and painkiller use. The use of semi-structured interviews allowed for the development of narratives that could sufficiently reflect the social and political context in which painkillers are consumed. All questions asked to participants were open-ended and sought to elicit narrative answers. This provided participants with ample opportunity to follow lines of thought that were not strictly directed by the researcher (Wengraf 2001). Follow-up questions, requests for more detail and reflection on the relevance to the research were developed informally throughout the interview session to more appropriately resemble the spontaneity of everyday conversation (Silverman 2013: 204). This approach provides the flexibility for the interviewee to contribute to the direction and content of the resulting data (Silverman 2013: 204).

Use of a conversational style is in deliberate response to the notion that the interview is a 'social event' (Hammersley and Atkinson 2007: 126) implicated in the constitutive production of the object of study (Law 2004). The specific wording of the questions thus changes with each interviewee, based variously on the language of the participant and the rapport developed with each person. Particular effort was made to adopt the language of the participant to keep the interview session conversational and relevant to the participant's own worldview (Rubin and Rubin 2012). This style avoids making the participant feel as though they are being interrogated by an authority figure. Interviews were thus also conducted in casual environments. Interviews took place in hotels (or Pubs) local to the participant, public parks, and coffee shops, as well as in private study rooms at various public libraries and at campuses of Western Sydney University. The more sensitive the information to be shared was likely to be, the more private a venue was sought. One interview was, for instance, conducted in the counseling room at Sydney's Medically Supervised Injecting Centre. In order to de-identify participants, names and other identifying details may have been removed or changed in the dissemination of data.

The sample of this study includes a mixed group of people that are derived from a diverse range of social and socioeconomic backgrounds. The diversity of the sample was spread across a range of demographic factors as well as the type and frequency of painkiller consumption. Majority of the sample was under the age of 40, with the mean age of the sample at 31. The gender spread was basically even, with 13 male participants and 12 female participants. Approximately half of the sample had completed high school to year 12, and a smaller group ($n = 6$) had undertaken tertiary education. The remainder of the sample had not completed high school (though 3 had completed high school equivalent qualification since leaving the traditional school system).

The research also targeted a board range of types and frequency of use among participants. Participants responded to advertisements targeting or self-identified with three broad categories such as aberrant/occasional use ($n = 8$), regular/recreational use ($n = 9$) and dependent use ($n = 8$). It is, however, also important to note that participants often discussed blurred boundary between these categories, and as such they were not used to guide the analysis processes.

These demographic and drug use practice groups were specifically targeted to both explore the qualitative features of the current set of practices being explore in the research and to expand the kinds of practices being observed. This approach allowed painkiller consumption and the practices that surrounded it to be placed in a broader context than only public health or criminal justice concerns. Analysis of the data acknowledges that participants have different relationships with painkillers in different contexts, making their effects and ways of use contextually contingent. One key feature of moving beyond dominant (medical) understandings of opiate consumption is a broader interpretation of the term dependence. The notion of being reliant on painkillers to maintain economic sustainability, emotional attachments or social relationships is used in conjunction with medical notions of tolerance and dependence. Forms of economic, emotional and social dependence are taken to be intimately related, rather than entirely separate to physical dependence on opiates.

Given that a variety of user perspectives form the empirical component of the project, it is also important to reflect on what the data collected represent in the context of this research. The interview data derived from conversations with participants should not be thought of as definitive descriptions of non-medical consumption. Neither should they be thought of as part of a holistically ethnographic description of how people practice the non-medical (ab)use of painkillers. The project demanded an acknowledgement that contradiction and contestation make up people's experiences of non-medical consumption. This means abandoning the notion that descriptions of such consumption can be neatly described as either 'accurate' or not. Silverman has noted that 'we need not hear interview responses simply as true or false reports on reality. Instead, we can treat such responses as displays of perspectives and moral forms' (1985: 157). In this way, information shared with the researcher represents stories about the lives of people who use pain medications, and the way they make sense of public and personal concerns about non-medical consumption.

The significance of narrative production is well established in cultural studies: 'People make sense of their experiences, claim identities, interact with each other, and participate in cultural conversations through storytelling' (Langellier and Peterson 2011: 1). The content of these interviews is thus used to analyze the social and political arrangements that participants deem to be part of the contexts in which they consume painkillers. The way in which participants describe those contexts, the language and phrasing they use, is also analyzed for the way it frames non-medical consumption within particular discourses.

Qualitative assessment of interview data is framed by a range of social theory about consumption and drug use in contemporary society that will be canvassed in the Part I and for which different aspects will be drawn out in Part II. The interview data presented in Part II begin an important qualitative framing of non-medical consumption absent from the current literature.

References

Acker, C. J. (2002). *Creating the American Junkie: Addiction Research in the Classic Era of Narcotic Control*. Baltimore and London: The Johns Hopkins University Press.

Alexander, A., & Roberts, M. S. (2012). *High Culture: Reflections on Addiction and Modernity*. Albany, NY: SUNY Press.

Bacchi, C. L. (2009). *Analysing Policy: What's the Problem Represented to Be?* Frenchs Forest: Pearson.

Barker, C., & Galasinski, D. (2001). *Cultural Studies and Discourse Analysis: A Dialogue on Language and Identity*. London: Sage.

Baudrillard, J. (1998). *The Consumer Society: Myths and Structures*. London: Sage.

Bauman, Z. (2001). *The Individualized Society*. New York: Wiley.

Bauman, Z. (2003). *Liquid Love: On the Frailty of Human Bonds*. New York: Wiley.

Bauman, Z. (2006). *Liquid Fear*. Cambridge: Polity Press.

Bauman, Z. (2007). *Liquid Times: Living in an Age of Uncertainty*. New York: Wiley.

Bauman, Z. (2013). *Liquid Life*. Cambridge: Wiley.
Beck, U. (1992). *Risk Society: Towards a New Modernity*. London: Sage.
Beck, U., Giddens, A., & Lash, S. (1994). *Reflexive Modernization: Politics, Tradition and Aesthetics in the Modern Social Order*. London, CA: Stanford University Press.
Becker, H. S. (1963).*Outsiders: Studies in the Sociology of Deviance*. London: Free Press of Glencoe.
Beckett, K. (1994). Setting the Public Agenda: "Street Crime" and Drug Use in American Politics. *Social Problems, 41*(3), 425–447.
Bell, S. E., & Figert, A. E. (2012). Medicalization and Pharmaceuticalization at the Intersections: Looking Backward, Sideways and Forward. *Social Science and Medicine, 75*(5), 775–783.
Benoit, C., Zadoroznyj, M., Hallgrimsdottir, H., Treloar, A., & Taylor, K. (2010). Medical Dominance and Neoliberalisation in Maternal Care Provision: The Evidence from Canada and Australia. *Social Science and Medicine, 71*(3), 475–481.
Blackett, T., & Robins, R. (2001). *Brand Medicine: The Role of Branding in the Pharmaceutical Industry*. Basingstoke: Palgrave Macmillan.
Blanch, B., Pearson, S., & Haber, P. S. (2014). An Overview of the Patterns of Prescription Opioid Use, Costs and Related Harms in Australia. *British Journal of Clinical Pharmacology, 78*(5), 1159–1166.
Bohnert, A. S. B., Valenstein, M., Bair, M. J., Ganoczy, D., McCarthy, J. F., Ilgen, M. A., et al. (2011). Association Between Opioid Prescribing Patterns and Opioid Overdose-Related Deaths. *Journal of the American Medical Association, 305*(13), 1315–1321.
Bourgois, P. (1995). *In Search of Respect: Selling Crack in El Barrio*. New York: Cambridge University Press.
Bowen, G. A. (2009). Document Analysis as a Qualitative Research Method. *Qualitative Research Journal, 9*(2), 27–40.
Bundy, H., & Quintero, G. (2017). From Mundane Medicines to Euphorigenic Drugs: How Pharmaceutical Pleasures are Initiated, Foregrounded, and Made Durable. *International Journal of Drug Policy, 49*, 109–116.
Burton, F., & Carlen, P. (2013). *Official Discourse (Routledge Revivals): On Discourse Analysis, Government Publications, Ideology and the State*. London: Taylor and Francis.
Campbell, N. D. (2007). *Discovering Addiction: The Science and Politics of Substance Abuse Research*. Ann Arbor: University of Michigan Press.

Carise, D., Dugosh, K. L., McLellan, A. T., Camilleri, A., Woody, G. E., & Lynch, K. G. (2007). Prescription OxyContin Abuse Among Patients Entering Addiction Treatment. *American Journal of Psychiatry, 164*(11), 1750–1756.

Carlson, R. G., Nahhas, R. W., Martins, S. S., & Daniulaityte, R. (2016). Predictors of Transition to Heroin Use among Initially Non-Opioid Dependent Illicit Pharmaceutical Opioid Users: A Natural History Study. *Drug Alcohol Dependence, 160,* 127–134.

Carney, M. (2010). *Oxy—The Hidden Epidemic. Four Corners.* Sydney: Australian Broadcasting Corporation.

Clarke, A. E., Shim, J. K., Mamo, L., Fosket, J. R., & Fishman, J. R. (2003). Biomedicalization: Technoscientific Transformations of Health, Illness, and US Biomedicine. *American Sociological Review, 68*(2), 161–194.

Coghlan, S., Gannoni, A., Goldsmid, S., Patterson, E., & Willis, M. (2015) *Drug Use Monitoring in Australia: 2013–14 Report on Drug Use Among Police Detainees* (AIC Reports, Monitoring Report 27). Canberra: Australian Ideal College.

Cohen, S. (1972). *Folk Devils and Moral Panics: The Creation of the Mods and Rockers.* London: MacGibbon and Kee.

Cohen, S., & Young, J. (1973). *The Manufacture of News: Social Problems, Deviance and the Mass Media.* London: Constable.

Coker, P., & Mackson, I. (2017). *Heroin(e).* Huntington, WV: TryBoro Productions and Nonstop Show Group.

Collison, M. (1996). In Search of the High Life: Drugs, Crime, Masculinities and Consumption. *British Journal of Criminology, 36*(3), 428–444.

Conrad, P. (2008). *The Medicalization of Society: On the Transformation of Human Conditions into Treatable Disorders.* Baltimore, MD: Johns Hopkins University Press.

Conrad, P., & Leiter, V. (2004). Medicalization, Markets and Consumers. *Journal of Health and Social Behavior, 45,* 158–176.

Conrad, P., & Schneider, J. W. (1980). *Deviance and Medicalization: From Badness to Sickness.* Philadelphia: Temple University Press.

Conrad, C., Bradley, H. M., Broz, D., Buddha, S., Chapman, E. L., Galand, R. R., et al. (2015). CommunityBaltimore Maryland Outbreak of HIV Infection Linked to Injection Drug Use of Oxymorphone—Indiana, 2015. *Morbidity and Mortality Weekly Report, 64*(16), 443–444.

Cooperstock, R. (1976). Psychotropic Drug Use among Women. *Canadian Medical Association Journal, 115*(8), 760.

Cooperstock, R. (1978). Sex Differences in Psychotropic Drug Use. *Social Science and Medicine, 12,* 179–186.
Dain, N. (1989). Critics and Dissenters: Reflections on "Anti-Psychiatry" in the United States. *Journal of the History of the Behavioral Sciences, 25*(1), 3–25.
Degenhardt, L., Knox, S., Barker, B., Britt, H., & Shakeshaft, A. (2005). Management of Alcohol, Tobacco and Illicit Drug Use Problems by General Practitioners in Australia. *Drug Alcohol Review, 24*(6), 499–506.
Degenhardt, L., Black, E., Breen, C., Bruno, R., Kinner, S., Roxburgh, A., et al. (2006). Trends in Morphine Prescriptions, Illicit Morphine Use and Associated Harms among Regular Injecting Drug Users in Australia. *Drug and Alcohol Review, 25*(5), 403–412.
Degrandpre, R. J., & White, E. (1996). Drug Dialectics. *Arena Journal, 7,* 41–63.
Duff, C. (2008). The Pleasure in Context. *International Journal of Drug Policy, 19*(5), 384–392.
Ehrenreich, B., & English, D. (1973). *Complaints and Disorders: The Sexual Politics of Sickness*. Old Westbury, NY: Feminist Press.
Ehrenreich, B., & English, D. (1978). *For Her Own Good: 150 Years of the Experts' Advice to Women*. Garden City, NY: Anchor Press.
Ferlie, E., McGivern, G., & FitzGerald, L. (2012). A New Mode of Organizing in Health Care? Governmentality and Managed Networks in Cancer Services in England. *Social Science and Medicine, 74*(3), 340–347.
Ferrell, J., & Stewart-Huidobro, E. (1996). *Crimes of Style: Urban Graffiti and the Politics of Criminality*. Boston, MA: Northeastern University Press.
Fischer, B., Bibby, M., & Bouchard, M. (2010). The Global Diversion of Pharmaceutical Drugs: Non-Medical Use and Diversion of Psychotropic Prescription Drugs in North America: A Review of Sourcing Routes and Control Measures. *Addiction, 105*(12), 2062–2070.
Fischer, B., Turnbull, S., Poland, B., & Haydon, E. (2004). Drug Use, Risk and Urban Order: Examining Supervised Injection Sites (SISs) as 'Governmentality'. *International Journal of Drug Policy, 15*(5–6), 357–365.
Fisher, M. A. (2003). Physicians and the Pharmaceutical Industry: A Dysfunctional Relationship. *Perspectives in Biology and Medicine, 46*(2), 254–272.
Foucault, M. (1973). *The Birth of the Clinic: An Archaeology of Medical Perception*. London: Routledge.
Foucault, M. (1988). *Madness and Civilisation: A History of Insanity in the Age of Reason*. New York, NY: Vintage Books.

Fraser, S. (2008). Trauma, Damage and Pleasure: Rethinking Problematic Drug Use. *International Journal of Drug Policy, 19*(5), 410–416.
Fraser, S., & Seear, K. (2013). *Making Disease, Making Citizens: The Politics of Hepatitis C.* Farnham: Ashgate Publishing.
Fraser, S., Moore, D., & Keane, H. (2014). *Habits: Remaking Addiction.* Basingstoke: Palgrave Macmillan.
Germov, J. (2009). *Second Opinion: An Introduction to Health Sociology.* South Melbourne: Oxford University Press.
Giddens, A. (1991). *Modernity and Self-Identity: Self and Society in the Late Modern Age.* Stanford, CA: Stanford University Press.
Hall, D. H., & Queener, J. E. (2007). Self-Medication Hypothesis of Substance Use: Testing Khantzian's Updated Theory. *Journal of Psychoactive Drugs, 39*(2), 151–158.
Hammersley, M., & Atkinson, P. (2007). *Ethnography: Principles in Practice.* London: Taylor and Francis.
Harris, G., Hodges, J. Q., & Snively, C. A. (2002). *OxyContin in Missouri: A Policy Brief Exploring Patterns of Abuse. Prevention, Treatment and Interdiction Strategies.* Columbia: Missouri Division of Alcohol and Drug Abuse, University of Missouri.
Hebdige, D. (1979). *Subculture: The Meaning of Style.* London: Methuen.
Hendler, R. A., Ramchandani, V. A., Gilman, J., & Hommer, D. W. (2013). Stimulant and Sedative Effects of Alcohol. In W. H. Sommer & R. Spanagel (Eds.), *Behavioral Neurobiology of Alcohol Addiction.* Berlin Heidelberg: Springer.
Holdcroft, A., Smith, M., Jacklin, A., Hodgson, H., Smith, B., Newton, M., et al. (1997). Pain Relief with Oral Cannabinoids in Familial Mediterranean Fever. *Anaesthesia, 52*(5), 483–486.
Holt, M., & Treloar, C. (2008). Pleasure and Drugs. *International Journal of Drug Policy, 19*(5), 349–352.
Holyfield, L., & Fine, G. A. (1997). Adventure as Character Work: The Collective Taming of Fear. *Symbolic Interaction, 20*(4), 343–363.
Horkheimer, M., Adorno, T. W., & Noerr, G. S. (1944). *Dialectic of Enlightenment: Philosophical Fragments.* Stanford, CA: Stanford University Press.
Hughes, J. (2008). *Pain Management: From Basics to Clinical Practice.* Rockville, MD: Elsevier.
Hunt, G. P., Evans, K., & Kares, F. (2007). Drug Use and Meanings of Risk and Pleasure. *Journal of Youth Studies, 10*(1), 73–96.

Illich, I. (1976). *Medical Nemesis: The Expropriation of Health*. New York: Pantheon Books.

Iversen, L., & Chapman, V. (2002). Cannabinoids: A Real Prospect for Pain Relief. *Current Opinion in Pharmacology, 2*(1), 50–55.

Jarvinen, M., & Ravn, S. (2011). From Recreational to Regular Drug Use: Qualitative Interviews with Young Clubbers. *Sociology of Health & Illness, 33*(4), 554–569.

Jonas, L. M. (1999). Making and Facing Danger: Constructing Strong Character on the River. *Symbolic Interaction, 22*(3), 247–267.

Jones, C. M., Logan, J., Gladden, R. M., & Bohm, M. K. (2015). Vital Signs: Demographic and Substance Use Trends Among Heroin Users—United States, 2002–2013. *Morbidity and Mortality Weekly Report, 64*(26), 719–725.

Keane, H. (2002). *What's Wrong With Addiction?* Melbourne: Melbourne University Press.

Keane, H., & Hamill, K. (2010). Variations in Addiction: The Molecular and the Molar in Neuroscience and Pain Medicine. *BioSocieties, 5*(1), 52–69.

Keane, H., Moore, D., & Fraser, S. (2011). Addiction and Dependence: Making Realities in the DSM. *Addiction, 106*(5), 875–877.

Kelly, P. (2005). *What is Liberalism?* Oxford: Polity.

Khantzian, E. J. (1997). The Self-Medication Hypothesis of Substance Use Disorders: A Reconsideration and Recent Applications. *Harvard Review of Psychiatry, 4*(5), 231–244.

Langellier, K., & Peterson, E. (2011). *Storytelling in Daily Life: Performing Narrative*. Philadelphia: Temple University Press.

Law, J. (2004). *After Method: Mess in Social Science Research*. London: Routledge.

Lende, D. H., Leonard, T., Sterk, C. E., & Elifson, K. (2007). Functional Methamphetamine Use: The Insider's Perspective. *Addiction Research & Theory, 15*(5), 465–477.

Lindesmith, A. R. (1938). A Sociological Theory of Drug Addiction. *American Journal of Sociology, 43*(4), 593–613.

Lupton, D. (1997). Foucault and the Medicalisation Critique. In R. Bunton & A. Petersen (Eds.), *Foucault, Health and Medicine*. London: Routledge.

Lupton, D. (2014). The Pedagogy of Disgust: The Ethical, Moral and Political Implications of Using Disgust in Public Health Campaigns. *Critical Public Health, 25*(1), 1–14.

Lyng, S. (2004). *Edgework: The Sociology of Risk-Taking*. London: Taylor and Francis.

Lyon, J. (2009). *Pill Head: The Secret Life of a Painkiller Addict*. New York: Hyperion.
Maher, L. (1997). *Sexed Work: Gender, Race, and Resistance in a Brooklyn Drug Market*. New York: Clarendon Press.
Markoua, A., Kostenb, T. R., & Koob, G. F. (1998). Neurobiological Similarities in Depression and Drug Dependence: A Self-Medication Hypothesis. *Neuropsychopharmacology, 18*(3), 135–174.
Marx, K. (1848). *The Communist Manifesto*. London: Bookmarks.
McCabe, S. E., West, B. T., Morales, M., Cranford, J. A., & Boyd, C. J. (2007). Does Early Onset of Non-Medical Use of Prescription Drugs Predict Subsequent Prescription Drug abuse and Dependence? Results from a National Study. *Addiction, 102*(12), 1920–1930.
Moore, D. (1993). Beyond Zinberg's 'Social Setting': A Processural View of Illicit Drug use. *Drug and Alcohol Review, 12*(4), 413–421.
Moore, D. (2004). Governing Street-Based Injecting Drug Users: A Critique of Heroin Overdose Prevention in Australia. *Social Science and Medicine, 59*(7), 1547–1557.
Moore, D. (2008). Erasing Pleasure from Public Discourse on Illicit Drugs: On the Creation and Reproduction of an Absence. *International Journal of Drug Policy, 19*(5), 353–358.
Moore, D., & Fraser, S. (2006). Putting at Risk What We Know: Reflecting on the Drug-Using Subject in Harm Reduction and its Political Implications. *Social Science and Medicine, 62*(12), 3035–3057.
Moore, D., & Valverde, M. (2010). Maidens at Risk: 'Date Rape Drugs' and the Formation of Hybrid Risk Knowledges. *Economy & Society, 25*(4), 514–531.
Nielsen, S., Larance, B., Bruno, R., Lintzeris, N., Vanderhaven, M., Lattas, G., et al. (2015). *Understanding the Health and Service Needs of Diverse Populations of Pharmaceutical Opioid Users: Cohort Studies of Dependent Users in Treatment, and People Who Inject Drugs*. Randwick: National Drug and Alcohol Research Centre, University of New South Wales.
O'Malley, P., & Valverde, M. (2004). Pleasure, Freedom and Drugs: The Uses of 'Pleasure' in Liberal Governance of Drug and Alcohol Consumption. *Sociology, 38*(1), 25–42.
Pearson, G. (1975). *The Deviant Imagination: Psychiatry, Social Work, and Social Change*. London: Macmillan.
Petersen, A., & Lupton, D. (1996). *The New Public Health: Health and Self in the Age of Risk*. Thousand Oaks, CA: Sage.

Petersen, A., Davis, M., Fraser, S., & Lindsay, J. (2010). Healthy Living and Citizenship: An Overview. *Critical Public Health, 20*(4), 391–400.

Phelan, J. C. (2005). Geneticization of Deviant Behavior and Consequences for Stigma: The Case of Mental Illness. *Journal of Health and Social Behavior, 46*(4), 307–322.

Race, K. (2009). *Pleasure Consuming Medicine: The Queer Politics of Drugs*. Durham, NC: Duke University Press.

Redfield, M., & Brodie, J. F. (2002). Introduction. In J. Farrell & M. Redfield (Eds.), *High Anxieties: Cultural Studies in Addiction*. Berkeley: University of California Press.

Reith, G. (2004). On the Edge: Drugs and the Consumption of Risk in Late Modernity. In S. Lyng (Eds.), *Edgework: The Sociology of Risk-Taking*. London: Taylor and Francis.

Rhodes, T. (2009). Risk Environments and Drug Harms: A Social Science for Harm Reduction Approach. *International Journal of Drug Policy, 20*(3), 193–201.

Rhodes, T., & Moore, D. (2001). On the Qualitative in Drugs Research: Part One. *Addiction Research & Theory, 9*(4), 279–297.

Rhodes, T., Singer, M., Bourgois, P., Friedman, S. R., & Strathdee, S. A. (2005). The Social Structural Production of HIV Risk Among Injecting Drug Users. *Social Science and Medicine, 61*(5), 1026–1044.

Ritzer, G. (2001). *Explorations in the Sociology of Consumption: Fast Food, Credit Cards and Casinos*. Thousand Oaks, CA: Sage.

Ritzer, G. (2005). *Enchanting a Disenchanted World: Revolutionizing the Means of Consumption*. Thousand Oaks, CA: Pine Forge Press.

Ritzer, G. (2014). *The McDonaldization of Society*. Thousand Oaks, CA: Sage.

Robson, P. (2009). *Forbidden Drugs*. Oxford: Oxford University Press.

Roxburgh, A., Bruno, R., Larance, B., & Burns, L. (2011). Prescription of Opioid Analgesics and Related Harms in Australia. *Medical Journal of Australia, 195*(5), 280–284.

Roxburgh, A., Hall, W. D., Dobbins, T., Gisev, N., Burns, L., Pearson, S., et al. (2017). Trends in Heroin and Pharmaceutical Opioid Overdose Deaths in Australia. *Drug and Alcohol Dependence, 179*, 291–298.

Rubin, H. J., & Rubin, I. S. (2012). *Qualitative Interviewing: The Art of Hearing Data*. Thousand Oaks, CA: Sage.

Rudd, R. A., Aleshire, N., Zibbell, J. E., & Gladden, R. M. (2016). Increases in Drug and Opioid Overdose Deaths—United States, 2000–2014. *American Journal of Transplantation, 16*(4), 1323–1327.

Salecl, R. (2004). *On Anxiety*. London: Routledge.
Saukko, P. (2003). *Doing Research in Cultural Studies: An Introduction to Classical and New Methodological Approaches*. Thousand Oaks, CA: Sage.
Seddon, T. (2006). Drugs, Crime and Social Exclusion: Social Context and Social Theory in British Drugs-Crime Research. *British Journal of Criminology, 46*(4), 680–703.
Silverman, D. (1985). *Qualitative Methodology and Sociology: Describing the Social World*. Aldershot: Gower.
Silverman, D. (2013). *Doing Qualitative Research: A Practical Handbook*. Thousand Oaks, CA: Sage.
Stein, M. (2009). *The Addict: One Patient, One Doctor, One Year*. New York: HarperCollins.
Sulkunen, P. (2002). Between Culture and Nature: Intoxication in Cultural Studies of Alcohol and Drug Use. *Contemporary Drug Problems, 29*, 253.
Szasz, T. S. (1961). *The Myth of Mental Illness: Foundations of a Theory of Personal Conduct*. New York: HarperCollins.
Szasz, T. S. (1970). *The Manufacture Of Madness: A Comparative Study of the Inquisition and the Mental Health Movement*. New York: Delta Book.
Taylor, I., Walton, P., & Young, J. (1973). *The New Criminology: For a Social Theory of Deviance*. London: Taylor and Francis.
Tunnell, K. D. (2005) The OxyContin Epidemic and Crime Panic in Rural Kentucky. *Contemporary Drug Problems, 32*(2), 225–258, 169–170.
Wazana, A. (2000). Physicians and the Pharmaceutical Industry: Is a Gift Ever Just a Gift? *Journal of the American Medical Association, 283*(3), 373–380.
Wengraf, T. (2001). *Qualitative Research Interviewing: Biographic Narrative and Semi-Structured Methods*. Thousand Oaks, CA: Sage.
Whelan, E., Asbridge, M., & Haydt, S. (2011). Representations of OxyContin in North American Newspapers and Medical Journals. *Pain Research & Management, 16*(4), 252–258.
White, W. L. (1998). *Slaying the Dragon: The History of Addiction Treatment and Recovery in America*. Bloomington, IL: Chestnut Health Systems.
Williams, S. J., Gabe, J., & Davis, P. (2008). The Sociology of Pharmaceuticals: Progress and Prospects. *Sociology of Health & Illness, 30*(6), 813–824.
Winlow, S., & Hall, S. (2006). *Violent Night: Urban Leisure and Contemporary Culture*. Oxford and London: Routledge.
Woolhose, M., Day, K., Rickett, B., & Milnes, K. (2012). 'Cos Girls Aren't Supposed to Eat Like Pigs Are They?' Young Women Negotiating Gendered Discursive Constructions of Food and Eating. *Journal of Health Psychology, 17*(1), 46–56.

Yokell, M. A., Delgado, M. K., Zaller, N. D., Wang, N., McGowan, S. K., & Green, T. (2014). Presentation of Prescription and Nonprescription Opioid Overdoses to US Emergency Departments. *Journal of the American Medical Association: Internal Medicine, 174*(12), 2034–2037.

Young, J. (1971). *The Drugtakers: The Social Meaning of Drug Use*. London: MacGibbon and Kee.

Zinberg, N. E. (1986). *Drug, Set, and Setting: The Basis for Controlled Intoxicant Use*. New Haven, CT: Yale University Press.

2

Drugs Through Time: The History of the Regulation of Drug Consumption in Australia

At the outset of the twentieth century, medical regulation and legal prohibition had not yet become a significant part of Australia's approach to 'drugs'. As such, there was little formal differentiation between legal and illegal opiates or medical and non-medical ways of consuming such substances. Today, opiates are tightly regulated through systems of international and domestic law, and their use is at the center of debates about health practice in most late-modern societies. These changes are often attributed to a growing awareness, both medical and scientific, of the harmful potential of particular opiates, with the emergence of what has been framed as a 'social problem' of significant concern. However, the social history of Australia's approach to drugs, and opiates in particular, paints a much more complex picture. This chapter traces the emergence of influential medical and political knowledge about drugs and its consequences for legislative regulation and health policy. Using a series of historical case studies, this chapter articulates how political knowledge and expert discourse have shaped the distinction between licit and illicit drugs.

Australian attitudes to drugs have always been highly influenced by the international context, and especially the policies and politics of the

G. C. Dertadian, *A Fine Line*,
https://doi.org/10.1007/978-981-13-1975-4_2

United States (US). The case studies covered in this chapter will therefore explore international events and movements to contextualize the way they have impacted Australian drug policy. The establishment of most Australian drug legislation has also been largely focused on opiates and other analgesics, which will thus form the basis of the historical investigation throughout the chapter.

Drawing on case studies between the start of the twentieth century to the present day, the chapter will articulate how distinctions between licit and illicit drugs have been shaped. It begins with a discussion of original drug legislation targeting 'opium suitable for smoking', the local policy influences of emerging American research interest in 'addiction' and the role of the medical profession and political establishment in regulating state-sanctioned forms of drug consumption. The chapter then goes on to explore how neoliberal economic policies have compounded the criminalizing effects of prohibitionist oriented drug legislation, as well as the US 'war on drugs' and its impacts on Australian policy and policing practice. Finally, the emergence of the harm minimization movement is discussed as an important example of contestation between models of medical and self-regulation.

'Opium Suitable for Smoking'

Established in the early twentieth century, some of the first laws restricting the use of drugs in Australia were aimed at 'opium suitable for smoking' (Brereton 2000). The reasons opium smoking was specifically 'targeted' in early drug legislation in North America and Europe are still contested in historical research. The Opium Wars of the nineteenth century are, however, a requisite starting point. Due to the culmination of diplomatic and trade disputes between the Chinese Quing Dynasty and the British Empire, the Opium Wars occurred between 1839–1842 and 1856–1860. It was during these periods that opium smoking was introduced into Chinese culture by the British. The smoking of opium was however viewed by the Chinese as a practice of the underclass (Hamilton et al. 1998). In North America the completion of the trans-America railroad in 1869 coincided with an influx of Chinese migrants in a time of recession, prompting a cultural backlash that included the vilification of opium smoking.

It was these political and economic conflicts, masked by issues of race, which eventually resulted in legislation about opium smoking in the early twentieth century. The international community played a key role in the development of early drug legislation in Australia, with the Commonwealth imposing an absolute ban on the importation of 'opium suitable for smoking' in 1905 (United Nations Office on Drugs and Crime 2008). Subsequently, State governments were pressured to introduce legislation criminalizing the manufacture, traffic, possession and use of 'opium suitable for smoking' (Carney 1981).

While there were important political and economic dimensions to the Opium Wars and the subsequent banning of opium smoking, the issue of race was central. For instance, similar legislation restricting opium use among Aboriginal people had already been implemented in Queensland's Aboriginals Protection and Restriction of the Sale of Opium Act 1897 (Purdie et al. 2010: 30). The legislation targeting opium smoking was also fundamentally racialized. This is because it targeted a form of drug consumption associated with Chinese migration, while ignoring the widespread use of other opium products that were popular among white Australians.

One of the most popular health products during the late ninetieth century and early twentieth century was called Laudanum, which was excluded from this early legislation. Widely used by white Australians, Laudanum was also known as Tincture of Opium. Perhaps the most infamous opiate-based drug, heroin, was also exempt. At the time heroin was a popular, easy to administer drug that was available without prescription (Duster 1970). Physicians of the time thought of heroin as being three times as potent as morphine, entirely non-addictive (Ray 1978), and an effective cure for 'opiate addiction': in fact "it was named Heroin for these 'heroic' properties" (Conrad and Leiter 2004: 121).

Though the pharmacology of opium smoking and the consumption of other opium-based products is largely identical, the practices were demographically distinct, leading many historians to observe the discriminatory nature of legislation targeting 'opium suitable for smoking' (Manderson 1988, 1999). In Australia, a significant element of opposition to opium smoking came from Chinese merchants, clergy-man and Chinese newspapers. Playing on the fears of 'White Australia', opposition to opium smoking often took on a sexual tone. Anxiety over keeping the 'purity' of White Australia perpetuated a perverted figure of the 'Chinaman', constantly depicted as a 'trafficker in young white women, and opium as the device by which the sexual inhibition or revulsion of young girls towards the Chinese could be trepanned, weak-ened, or overborne' (Manderson 2005: 45). During the late nineteenth century, there were a number of reports commissioned by various gov-ernment bodies which sought to "give some idea of the prevalence of vice and depravity induced by this enslaving and degrading practice" (Sydney City & Suburban Sewage and Health Board 1875–1876).

Antagonism toward opium smoking was not limited to Chinese newspapers. Anti-Chinese sentiment informed an entire policy agenda during the early twentieth century, with opium smoking forming what Manderson refers to as one "tentacle of the octopus" (Manderson 1993: 15). Perhaps the most significant example of racialized government pol-icy included the restrictions placed on Chinese immigration, like those found in the Immigration Restriction Act 1855 (Vic), the Chinese Restriction and Regulation Act 1888 (NSW) and the Immigration Restriction Act 1901 (Cth). Discriminatory immigration legislation was often justified on the grounds of the financial security of white miners (Lake and Reynolds 2008).

As part of a push from the Chinese elite, and a social anxiety about maintaining 'White Australia', a range of discriminatory government pol-icies were introduced in the early twentieth century (Dyster and Meredith 1990) that sought to deter aspects of Chinese culture within Australian migrant communities. Part of this series of discriminatory policies included legislation about the smoking of opium because it was associated with the Chinese population. A web of politically motivated, racialized discourses informed shifting approaches to drug regulation in Australia. Legislation targeting practices common among Chinese migrants reveals little scientific motivation for early legislative structures to regulate opium. Instead, such legislation illustrates the influence of political forces that have long informed 'official' distinctions between kinds of opiates, the way they are consumed and the people who consume them.

Addiction, Medicine and Drug Policy

Another driving force behind the push for Australian policy makers to regulate opiates was the emergence of 'addiction' in American research. During the 1920s, some of the earliest research on the physiology of addiction was conducted on monkey colonies ('junkie monkeys'). Campbell has noted that these research subjects were purposefully chosen as they were best positioned to perform a version of drug dependence that appealed to US funding bodies of the time. In order to avoid the perceived pitfalls of researching the pleasurable aspects of drug use, researchers "turned to animal models both to bracket desire and to place their research on the more objective ground sought by the NRC [National Research Council] Committee on Drug Addiction" (Campbell 2007: 29). Psychiatric research with prison populations in the 1920s and 1930s also appealed to the NRCs investment in 'drug addiction' as a criminal pathology.

The work of psychiatrist Lawrence Kolb played an important role in the development of early twentieth-century medical models of 'drug addiction'. Among a set of six addict 'types', Kolb formulated a distinction between 'normal persons who have become addicted accidentally or... through medical treatment" and people who have "immature, hedonistic, socially inadequate personality' (Kolb 1962: 5–6). The moralizing implication of distinguishing between 'normal' people who were the victims of medical misconduct and 'psychopaths' who were motivated by a hedonistic pursuit of pleasure has had a lasting impact in the addictions field. Kolb's later work with prisoners at a facility in Lexington Kentucky, infamously known as the Lexington Narcotic Farm, also reinforced the notion that there is a clear distinction between the physiological and psychological elements of addiction.

The prominence of the physiological/psychological distinction in psychiatric research was partly a reflection of the notion that at the time, addiction was largely thought of as an iatrogenic condition. Latrogenesis traditionally refers to situations in which a patient has been harmed in the process of medical treatment or as a result of the negligence of a medical practitioner—iatrogenic addiction is "addiction caused in the course of medical treatment" (Acker 2002: 29–30). Based on the assumption that most 'normal' people could be protected if opiate use in medical treatment was restricted, the psychiatric community advocated for expansions to the US Harrison Act 1914, a piece of legislation originally designed to regulate and record the supply of opiates.

Kolb's work on addiction and crime in the 1920s advocated that 'drug addiction' was a medical problem, and that treatment, not law enforcement was the solution. However, in the looming shadow of alcohol prohibition the American political climate was veering toward the banning of drugs. Expansions to the Harrison Act 1914 during 1920s and 1930s meant that the act became increasingly punitive (Conrad and Scheider 1980: 124–125). Though Kolb and others in the psychiatric community advocated for a medical response to 'drug addiction', support for the expansion of the Harrison Act 1914 meant that, ironically, psychiatry played an important part in the institutional criminalization of addiction.

The criminalization of addiction in the US also had an influence on the way medical practitioners related to the 'addict' population. During the 1930s and 1940s, the American Medical Association was closely monitoring changes to the Harrison Act 1914 and had been vocal about its opposition to provisions that diminished the authority of the medical profession—through restrictions on medical authority to prescribe opiates. As a consequence of judicial interpretations of the Harrison Act 1914 which were becoming increasingly punitive, the demographic of 'opiate addicts' was shifting to be more clearly associated with young inner-city men who were increasingly seen as 'deviant' thrill seekers (Conrad and Schneider 1980).

As the only profession to have legitimate access to opiates, the prescribing physicians became the only legal avenue to acquire the drugs that 'addicts' required. Throughout the 1930s and 1940s, sections of the medical profession became increasingly frustrated by having to act as gatekeeper to the 'thrill-seeker's drug:

> physicians became increasingly wary of patients complaining of mysterious pains and demanding relief through drugs. As addicts became undesirable patients, the motivation to study the physiological mechanisms or human dimensions of addiction waned. (Acker 2002: 62)

With the institutional criminalization of addiction, there was an increasing distance between the medical profession and the 'addict population' of the US. A growing number of people dependent on opiates began to turn to, and eventually depend on, illicit markets for the supply of drugs like heroin (Conrad and Schneider 1980: 127). As a result, stigmatized images of the urban 'junkie' proliferated in American society throughout the middle of the twentieth century.

International frameworks for medical models of addiction echoed aspects of the American context. In 1957, the World Health Organization (WHO) published a series of definitions relating to substance use. The first, addiction, emphasized the need for both physical and psychological dependence and the second, habituation, placed emphasis on only psychological dependence (Zinberg 1986: 29–30). The distinction between 'addiction' and 'habituation' reinforced the notion that people who have become drug dependent because of recreational drug use were the 'real addicts'. In 1964, the WHO abandoned the term 'addiction' for 'drug dependence', though its definition still emphasizes an implicitly moral distinction between the physiological and the psychological aspects of addiction (Keane and Hamill 2010: 55). These formulations of addiction and related terms link closely with psychiatric research by Kolb and others who followed in a similar tradition. At the international level, the physiological/psychological distinction functioned as justification for the demonization of drugs like heroin and the stigmatization of people who use it.

As a young nation, Australia was often influenced by developments in the international community. After the implementation and expansion of the Canadian Opium and Drug Act 1911, the British Dangerous Drugs Act 1920 and the American Harrison Act 1914, international pressure was mounting for Australia to implement similar policies of criminalization. The Commonwealth intervened to impose further restrictions on the importation of opium (as well as other drugs including cocaine, marijuana, etc.), and State governments followed in similar fashion with laws criminalizing heroin possession and use throughout the 1920s. Yet by the 1930s Australia was still "using 7.5 per cent of the world's legal [medically prescribed] heroin supply'" (Rowe 2005: 108), which amounted to approximately three times that of the British (per capita) and nearly fifty times that of the United States (per capita) (Rolfe 1989). However, most of these prescriptions were for people who were dependent on opiates, and if the British and American contexts allow any insight, much of the 'addict' population at the time was still white, middle-aged housewives and doctors (Conrad and Schneider 1980).

Unlike their American counterparts, Australian physicians continued to medically maintain people dependent on heroin well into the 1950s. While Australia lingered behind other developed nations in the banning of heroin, the Australian medical profession did place intense focus on reducing and regulating the 'non-medical use' of heroin throughout the first half of the twentieth century. Advocacy for the medicalization of 'addiction' ensured that the medical profession could gain greater control over the prescription of heroin:

> …by defining all users of illegal drugs [such as heroin] as addicts, breaking the law itself became a sign of illness. Medical authority was therefore entrenched… the medical user had already acknowledged medical power, and the non-medical user was sick by definition, and was therefore an appropriate subject of medical intervention… [and] legal controls. (Manderson 1993: 103)

What was considered 'proper use' of heroin was increasingly left to the discretion of the medical expert, and the 'addict' label fostered an increasing convergence between the medical and legal control of people who use opiates in Australia.

The Role of Medical and Political Involvement

For the first hundred years of Australian history since colonization, drugs seemed to be an issue of very little significance to policy makers. The development of foundational frameworks for Australian drug legislation was mostly produced in response to international pressure (Lupton and Najman 1995). With the growing influence of British and particularly American conservative and Temperance movements in the nineteenth and early twentieth century, the regulation of the world's drug supply became a staple of international policy transfers and law (Levine 1993; Sulkunen and Warpenius 2000). Tension between the passionate international pursuit of drug regulation and Australian ambivalence to the issue meant that Australia repeatedly gave into international pressure as drugs were too inconsequential an issue to risk the country's international standing (Manderson 1993).

While drug policy was initially accorded little significance by Australian lawmakers, its introduction did require a governing group of professionals to function as regulators. During the early twentieth century, there were three main competing sellers of drug products: doctors, druggists (who were representatives of the patent medicine industry) and pharmacists. Rapid advances in medical science were among the most important factors involved in the rise of the medical profession as the foremost 'legitimate' provider of drugs. By the 1920s in the US and abroad, 'hygienic successes over germ-borne illness ushered in a new era of medicine that addressed chronic, non-infectious ailments including heart disease, kidney disease, and cancer' (Nadesan 2008: 107). As developments in the addictions field demonstrate, the medical profession was the unequivocal victor in the right to regulate drugs. The growing influence of medicine meant that medical knowledge was also becoming more specialized. A new division of labor in the medical profession meant that dentists, midwives and nurses, among others, became marginalized members of the medical community (Willis 1989).

As the medical community gradually gained prescriptive authority over more and more substances, druggists and the patent medicine industry dissipated, while pharmacists were relegated to a dispensary role (Manderson 1993). Moreover, by the 1940s the medical profession had not only won the authority to regulate drugs, but perhaps more significantly had become culturally accepted as the ultimate arbiter of physical and mental health (Freidson 1988). It was in this context that perhaps the most significant movement in social and political approaches to drugs occurred.

Legal heroin use in Australia almost doubled in the mid- to late 1940s from the already high rates of the 1930s. This increase prompted international concern about Australia's attitude to heroin from the United Nations, and more particularly the US. Borrowing almost exclusively from the rhetoric of American proponents of prohibition, calls to ban the use of heroin, medically or otherwise, became more and more prominent in Australia. Despite no recorded deaths by heroin overdose in Australia between 1943 and 1953 (Wodak and Owens 1996), and opposition from sections of the medical profession (Rowe 2005), lawmakers placed a complete ban on heroin in 1953. The ban effectively criminalized everyone who had been using heroin at the time and the doctors who medically maintained their supply, while also guaranteeing the expansion of the criminal networks that had already emerged in response to tightening regulations. Similar bans on cocaine, marijuana and the like followed (Brereton 2000).

By the 1960s, Australian states were still complying with international pressure through increased sanctions, but for the first time they were doing so without objection. Politicians and bureaucrats started to see the potential for prestige and power in drug regulation, and, for the first time in Australian history lawmakers were behaving as if drugs mattered: 'politicians saw votes in it, bureaucrats saw power and prestige in its administration' (Manderson 1993: 141). A newfound interest in building a structure of Australian drug regulation saw a convergence of the interests of the medical profession and government bureaucracies. This allowed for medical authority to inform a socially constructed distinction between 'licit' medical opiates (analgesic medications) and 'illicit' recreational opiates (heroin). The formulation of 'addiction' and its impact on drug policy is one important example of the impact of the overlapping interests of medical and political authority during the middle of the twentieth century. These overlapping interests also had consequences for the regulation of other drugs, such as alcohol.

The Six O'Clock Swill

The fact that there was now political capital to be gained through public condemnation of drugs began to inform considerable transformations in the social significance of particular drugs, and those who used them.

Since the early twentieth century, alcohol had been the largest target of campaigns against the 'moral ills' of inebriate consumption. It was in this time that the Australian Temperance movement shifted from their long-standing position (since the 1830s) of advocating moderation to a strong lobbying effort for alcohol prohibition, which 'at times came surprisingly close to success' (Manderson 1993: 51). The vigor of Temperance campaigns for alcohol prohibition is at least partly thought to be reflective of the role alcohol played in domestic violence (Leonard 2002).

Following influential campaigns from Temperance movements, South Australia voted, in a referendum in 1916, for six o'clock closing times for pubs and hotels (Phillips 1980). New South Wales, Victoria and Tasmania followed suit the very next year. The implications of the policy change were not, however, particularly congenial to the agendas of alcohol abstinence and prohibition. The new closing time initiated an exponential climb in alcohol consumption in the hour leading up to 6 p.m. The rush to get to the pub after finishing work and to consume as much as possible before it closed became a common part of Australian drinking culture, infamously known as the 'six o'clock swill'.

Faced with the tightening regulation of opiates and other drugs toward the middle part of the century, the powerful influence of Temperance movements and their conservative hold over alcohol regulation began to fade (Blocker et al. 2003). The long-standing popularity of six o'clock closing times for bars and hotels soon began to wane (Phillips 1980). By the 1950s, NSW had moved to ten o'clock closing times, and Victoria and South Australia followed in the 1960s. With the decline of Australian Temperance movements, alcohol consumption became less associated with the determined drunkenness of the era of the six o'clock swill (Room 2010).

As Australia moved into the second half of the twentieth century, the medical profession also cooperated in the process of deregulating and destigmatizing alcohol. References to alcoholism were increasingly deployed in medical research and public discourse, purposefully separating alcohol dependence from other, more stigmatized forms of addiction; alcohol was considered safe, and it was the individual alcoholic who was the problem (Levine 1978). Soon women also began to be reintroduced into mainstream cultures of public drinking and by the 1960s alcohol started to be associated with sports, recreation and dining out.

In the face of a complete ban on many drugs previously used as intoxicants, alcohol seemed to form a new state-sanctioned outlet for inebriation (Fitzgerald and Jordan 2011). This made way for the further stigmatization and marginalization of those now firmly deemed 'illicit drug users' and 'drug addicts'. Due in part to the increased regulation of drugs, a deep division between legal medical use and illegal non-medical 'abuse' began to emerge in the social milieu of Australian culture. Drugs that occupied the wrong side of this divide were now commonly, though often misleadingly, referred to as 'narcotics'. These newly termed narcotics and those who consumed them were considered to embody the antithesis of good sense and social responsibility. By the 1960s, 'drugs' simply did not signify a single, unified cultural meaning anymore. Heroin was no longer just a 'drug', but a narcotic as well; alcohol was no longer a drug at all, rather it was a drink; cigarettes became smokes; morphine became medicine.

The Pharmaceutical Benefits Scheme

The introduction of the Pharmaceutical Benefits Scheme (PBS) in 1948 is another key example of the way medical and government regulation had become intimately intertwined. As Australia moved into the second half of the twentieth century, its political and bureaucratic systems of drug regulation relied increasingly on the medical profession.

During his Prime Ministership (1945–1949), Ben Chifley embarked on an ambitious campaign to create a British-style National Health Service for Australia. As part of this campaign in 1948, Chifley introduced the PBS. In its early incarnations, the PBS was a limited scheme which provided 139 "lifesaving and disease preventing" drugs free of charge to pensioners and others in the community (Commonwealth of Australia 2013). Most of Chifley's health reforms were eventually ruled unconstitutional by the High Court of Australia, with the exception of the PBS. Established in 1953 the Pharmaceutical Benefits Advisory

Committee (PBAC) decided what pharmaceuticals would be included in the government's Formulary, and thus what was available under the PBS. The PBAC eventually became an independent statutory body under the National Health Act 1953, mostly comprised of members of the medical profession.

By 1960, the PBS had been expanded and nominal user charges began to be applied. The benefits of more affordable medications were politically resonant and continued to gain popularity. The 1970s saw large-scale increases in the products available on the PBS, and the government expenditure accompanying it (Biggs 2002). As expenditure grew so did the nominal charges that were applied to the medications. Still, it was not until the mid-1980s that patient contributions were significantly increased to offset the major expenditure that the PBS now represented. Since its implementation, each government had expanded the PBS program, further entrenching the cultural distinctions between legal and illegal drugs. Perhaps more importantly though, the PBS formed part of a wider process of normalizing the consumption of pharmaceuticals in medical treatment (Crawford 1980) and the medicalization of Australian society fueled the expansion of the PBS.

The trend of medicalization and increases in pharmaceutical intervention were also occurring in other developed nations with established traditions of Western medicine. Observations about medicalization and the growth of 'pill culture' were prominent in North America and the UK (Hogshire and Alfvegren 1999; Jackson 1966; Miles 1953). The consumption of pills was becoming a common part of everyday life for most developed nations. For Australians, this global trend was being legitimized by expansions to the PBS.

By the time nominal charges to the PBS had increased significantly in the 1980s, pharmaceuticals had been a staple of the developed world for decades, and their subsidization in Australia for nearly as long meant that their use had become deeply normalized. The expansion of the PBS during the second half of the twentieth century reinforced medical authority and the growing perception of 'safety' attached to the medications available on its formulary. The similarities with the state-sanctioning of alcohol discussed in the previous section are salient. The removal of barriers to alcohol consumption and the subsidization of pharmaceuticals seemed to permissively condone the consumption of these drugs, at least in comparison with illicit drugs.

'A Cup of Tea, a Bex, and a Good Lie Down'

The consumption of over-the-counter headache powders forms an important part of the legacy of the normalization of pharmaceuticals and the medicalization of pain in Australian history. Prior to the introduction of the PBS, analgesic powder medications had been very popular in Australia. As far back as 1907, one observer points out 'What the drink habit is to men in Australia, the headache powder is among women' (Murray 1980: 9). Products such as Bex and Vincent's powders were over-the-counter analgesics recommended for the treatment of minor aches and pains. Bex and Vincent's powders contained, as their main ingredients, a combination of aspirin, phenacetin and caffeine (APC), and were used as a cure for low moods, a remedy to help calm you down, and a painkiller. During the 1950s, Australia became the largest consumer of over-the-counter analgesics in the world, particularly APCs (Shelley 1967).

Due to the high levels of APC consumption during the 1950s there was a sharp increase in chronic gastric ulceration (Billington 1960; Billington 1963) and kidney failure (Kincain-Smith 1969) in women in particular—the condition became known as analgesic nephropathy (Stelle et al. 1969). However, the medical community in Australia resisted the notion that legally available medications like Bex and Vincent's could be implicated in the increase in gastrointestinal complications and kidney failure (Murray 1980). The divide between legal and illegal drugs, which the medical profession was instrumental in establishing, implied that those who were legally obtaining their drugs should not be condemned. The illegal drug users, it was thought, were the 'real problem' (Manderson 1993).

Reluctance to acknowledge the connection between increased consumption of APCs and medical complications was clearly tied to the now entrenched cultural assumption that legal medications were 'safe' and illegal drugs were 'dangerous'. During the middle of the twentieth century, many Australians used APCs regularly (Stewart 1978), some daily, and trepidation to confront the complications associated with APC consumption was linked to a reluctance to undermine the safe/dangerous drug dynamic. In a 1980 publication in the British Journal of Addiction, Murray observes that:

> Not only was there reluctance to admit that everyday medicines like aspirin and phenacetin could cause kidney damage, but there was also resistance to the idea that the drugs were being taken for other than medical reasons. (Murray 1980: 10)

It has also been argued that APCs were a mechanism for the continued domestic control of women who felt unhappy in the 1950s:

> As a cure-all for women who felt unwell or depressed, 'a Bex and a good lie down' was an Australian cultural tradition. It was a way to suppress women's feelings of alienation, an agency of their oppression, and an easy means of social control. (Manderson 1993: 136)

With the combination of a threat to the social order and the promise of the continued domestic control of women, the status quo surrounding the safety of over-the-counter medications—APCs in particular—was firmly cemented in Australian culture throughout the 1950s.

It was not until the 1960s that the medical profession formally acknowledged the link between analgesic nephropathy and the use of APCs. Subsequently the early 1960s saw a slight decrease in the importation of phenacetin into Australia (Hennessey 1993). However, medical evidence linking APC consumption and gastrointestinal and kidney complications was still limited. In an attempt to explain away the issue, excessive APC consumption became presented as a 'female problem'. Largely as a result of the growing influence of psychology, an increasing number of undesirable and socially unacceptable behaviors exhibited by women were being diagnosed (or rather misdiagnosed) as symptoms of 'hysteria' (Hennessey 1992). In an article published in the Annals of Internal Medicine in 1968, the authors describe the 'typical' analgesic nephropathy patient as a female whose:

> life history reveals a broken home, an early short-lived marriage, and frequent loss of time from work due to illness. She suffers from insomnia, takes sedatives, and a few years ago took an overdose. She complains, tearfully of weakness, indigestion, and recent vomiting. Most oppressive are her headaches which she has had for twenty years, but which have become virtually continuous and are driving her to thoughts of suicide. Her medical history is lengthy and includes neurological, haematological, psychiatric, and gastro-intestinal evaluations. She was hospitalised for depression and five years ago had a gastrectomy for a bleeding pepticulcer. (Gault et al. 1968: 14)

The representation of APC consumption as a 'female problem' invisibilized the wider circumstances which drove women to take power analgesics and the specific pharmacological imperatives that kept women dependent on the drug.

In Australia, the 1950s were a time of contradiction for many women, where changing dynamics, domestic responsibilities and marital commitments were in constant conflict. Women were forced back into domesticity after the male population returned from the Second World War. While some women seemed to welcome the change, many others felt the boredom of domestic living was unbearable in comparison with the excitement of the working world (Hartman 1978). The increase in childbirth during the 'baby boom' era meant women's domestic responsibility grew with the amount of children they had (Burnley 1982). Speedy advances in technology were thought to make housework quicker and less demanding; however, the standard of cleanliness was now raised substantially, and a greater focus was placed on women to remain youthful and physically attractive (Hennessey 1992).

By the 1960s, the amount of married women in the workforce had grown substantially, yet women's work was still mostly considered unimportant. Hennessey writes that:

> despite growing community recognition that many women were finding it increasingly difficult to cope with the demands placed on them, the cause of their stress and tension was not perceived as overwork. Rather it was diagnosed as personal inadequacy, more a function of being a woman than a product of women's work. (1992: 260)

The circumstances of women's lives were left out of the equation in medical accounts about APC consumption.

The medical community focused its resources on isolating the nephrotoxic properties of APCs, while ignoring their energy-boosting components and the potential for people to become dependent on them. Professor Priscilla Kincaid's work on analgesic nephropathy was influential as it leads to the discovery that the combination of aspirin and phenacetin was most damaging (Australian Academy of Science 2013). However, it was not until the late 1960s that Kincaid's discoveries became well known among the medical community, and not until the late 1970s that legislation was introduced to control the combination of aspirin and phenacetin in over-the-counter analgesics.

The effects of caffeine on those consuming APCs were also largely ignored until the 1970s. As a major component of APCs, caffeine is a central nervous system stimulant that provided the energy that women of the time needed to meet the growing demands placed on them. The regular consumption of caffeine creates a steadily increasing tolerance, which meant that women were taking more and more Bex and Vincent's powders to get the same burst of energy. Both the excessive consumption of and withdrawal from caffeine induces the kind of headaches that so many women of the time complained of. Knowledge of caffeine headaches was available to the medical community in Australia since at least the 1940s (Dreisbach and Pfeiffer 1943), and yet at the time women's headaches were still mostly dismissed as symptoms of hysteria.

This meant that women were steadily increasing their dose of APCs to get the same energy-boosting effects, while at the same time the amount of caffeine intake was inducing headaches, which were dismissed as symptoms of neurosis. Due to caffeine withdrawal, any attempt to stop using APCs only made the headaches worse. In among this vicious cycle, women were first told that the drugs they were consuming were entirely safe, then safe in moderation, then, once a nation of women were thoroughly dependent, that their compulsive consumption was a symptom of psychiatric dysfunction and personal inadequacy.

This controversy is an important instance of the medicalization of pain in Australian society. The desire to medicate physical pain alongside emotional difficultly is also an important part of the controversy. Another key element is the historical conditions that established a perceived 'safety' around pharmaceuticals. It is this impression of safety that informed the medical profession's reluctance to acknowledge and its slow response to the harmful effects of APCs, as well as the ease with which most women took to the use of such medications. The remainder of this chapter addresses the other component of the safe/dangerous drug dynamic: drugs thought to be 'harmful' and 'dangerous'. It deals with trends in Western approaches to social welfare, as well as the emergence of 'war on drugs' rhetoric and harm minimization policy.

Neoliberalism and the 'War on Drugs'

The harms associated with illicit drug use are often presented as being caused by the properties of the drug or the choices of its consumer, while the political economy that informs problematic consumption is often relegated to the background. The history of opiate regulation, alcohol consumption and pharmaceutical and analgesic use outlined above illustrate the limitations of assuming pharmacology and psychology determine the harms of drugs use. A growing chorus of sociological, anthropological and public health research (Bourgois 2002) has demonstrated that a focus on the pharmacology of the drug and the psychology of the consumer over-determines their role in the uptake of 'risky' or 'harmful' drug-taking practices (Zinberg 1986). Economic and social welfare policies are in fact central to the potential harms of drug use. This section elaborates on how the formation of political approaches to welfare and social support has changed in advanced liberal economies over the last century, the links this has to the establishment of the 'War on Drugs', and its impacts on policy and policing practice in Australia.

In the context of the US Great Depression during the early 1930s, a series of monetary policies between 1933 and 1936, dubbed 'the new deal', provided financial support for and government intervention into struggling industries so that levels of employment could be stabilized. The importance of reducing unemployment came to inform a wider philosophy about the role of the state in economic management.

A political philosophy about the role of the economy in ensuring the welfare of all citizens was subsequently developed. Termed 'embedded liberalism' this approach has been briefly summarized as requiring that:

> the state should focus on full employment, economic growth, and the welfare of its citizens, and that state power should be freely deployed, alongside of or, if necessary, intervening in or even substituting for market processes to achieve these ends. (Harvey 2005: 10)

Embedded liberalism was both a political and economic philosophy that placed social welfare above the accumulation of individual wealth. The proliferation of embedded liberalism throughout global economic policy, especially during the middle of the twentieth century, produced high rates of economic growth in modern capitalist economies.

However, by the late-1960s and 1970s the effectiveness of embedded liberalism began to collapse. Capitalist economies started showing signs of over-accumulation, and a related devaluing of capital investment. During the 1970s, the world entered a phase of stubbornly stagnated inflation (or 'stagflation') that set the scene for a deliberate project by the wealthiest elements of the developed world to begin to introduce, what has come to be known as neoliberal economic policy (Harvey 2005). Pursued by influential corporate and conservative interests, neoliberalism began as a political philosophy about the liberation of individual entrepreneurialism through frameworks of deregulated (or free) markets and trade. Though it emerged in uneven ways across the globe, its influence in economic policy has become widespread.

Harvey (2005) has noted that a series of key political and policy events during the late 1970s and early 1980s mark the start of 'the neoliberal turn'. Since then the 'free market' mentality has formed part of a larger philosophy about limiting the role of government in order to unleash the entrepreneurial potential of the individual. The spread of neoliberal thought has contributed to the remaking of the modern condition in disparate areas such as 'divisions of labor, social relations, welfare provisions, technological mixes, ways of life and thought, reproductive activities, attachments to the land and habits of the heart' (Harvey 2005: 2). However, the liberalization of drug regulation was exempt from the neoliberal interest in individual freedom, largely because neoliberalism was associated with conservative elements within the political system that had traditionally championed drug prohibition.

As the 'Western world' moved into the second half of the twentieth century, unequal access to the ideals of modern consumerism (Young 2011) and reduced investment in social support (Reiner 2012) were exacerbating the criminalizing imperative of drug legislation in advanced liberal economies. Class interests seeking a reduction in government intervention into the accumulation of individual wealth seized upon the international trend of stagflation during the 1960s and 1970s as an opportunity to erode popular consensus about the social welfare and social democratic role of the state.

This period saw unprecedented increases in drug use and associated drug convictions (Gahlinger 2004). Strong links have since been developed between neoliberal policies and the development of what is often termed problem drug use (Punch 2005; Room 2005; Singer 2008). Increased levels of income inequality are an identifiable consequences of neoliberal economic management (Baer and Maloney 1997; Navarro 2007), which has contributed to a range of adverse health outcomes, with harmful drug use high among the list (De Vogli 2011; Galea et al. 2003; Wilkinson et al. 2003). America's 'war on drugs' has played into aspects of the erosion of traditional liberal approaches to welfare and social support.

In 1968, Richard Nixon won the US Presidency on the promise that he would 'restore law and order', drawing in particular on the issue of drug control. In 1972, President Nixon declared a 'total war against dangerous drugs', launching the term 'war on drugs' into the popular vernacular. Domestically, Nixon's war on drugs was simply a continuation of already well-established prohibitionist policy. However, as a result of a sharper focus on the issue, partly through the creation of the new Drug Enforcement Agency (DEA), an increase in drug-related convictions meant the prison system began to fill at unprecedented rates (Gahlinger 2004).

The establishment of a war on drugs also had implications for the international community, particularly as Nixon had begun to emphasize that the supply of 'dangerous substances' were from international sources. Nixon represented the 'drug problem' as a foreign threat to the American (and 'Western') way of life. Supply reduction, enforced through the threat of international embargoes and other forms of often militarized hostility, became the centerpiece of international drug policy. Australian drug policy never formally adopted a 'war on drugs', but it did incorporate significant aspects of US drug policy and law enforcement at the time.

The introduction of an American war on drugs, and its implications around the world, had a transformative impact on the political climate of the 1970s. In response to the defiance of countercultural drug cultures, concern about the physical dangers of illegal drugs gave way to concern over their 'social impact'. References to narcotics were being replaced with discussion about the 'misuse' and 'abuse' of drugs. Race observes that concern about drug use during the 1970s and 1980s were 'no longer [about] the scientific properties of specific substances, nor the physical dangers arising from their consumption' (2005). Instead, concern began to surround "the character of their use [and] its deviation from [the] professional authority, that form[ed] the locus of juridical consideration" (Race 2005).

Medical authority once again emerged as important in defining the acceptable use of a drug, and thus also what constituted its 'misuse'. A move toward a language of 'misuse' and 'abuse' cemented the impression of social deviance that had been engendered by the medical profession throughout the century. However, in contrast to previous bans on opium smoking, the 'war on drugs' did not focus on 'proper' or 'improper' forms of consumption, but rather on the legal status of a drug itself. Any consumption of an illicit drug was considered non-medical and thus constituted 'misuse' and/or 'abuse' (Manderson 1995; Race 2005).

Australia continued to follow trends in drug enforcement throughout the 1970s with the ratification of a range of international treaties relating to drugs, including the Convention on Psychotropic Substances 1971 and the Protocol Amending the Single Convention 1972. These conventions provided limited recognition of the disappointing progress of the international model of prohibition, calling for more attention to health and social outcomes (Miller 2009). Despite this, the international community remained committed to the supply and demand reduction approaches that had been reinvigorated by a devolving of the importance of the social welfare function of the State.

During the 1970s, the Commonwealth implemented the Customs Amendment Act No. 2 1971 (Cwlth), which made the traffic of a 'drug of addiction' a separate offence. Following this Commonwealth legislation, the Poisons (Amendment) Act 1970 (NSW) brought NSW up to speed with its state counterparts by making it a separate offence to sell or deal a 'drug of addiction' (Manderson 1993). Where it was once a criminal offence to be in possession of an illegally imported substance, it now became an offence to possess any narcotic 'reasonably suspected' of being illegally imported. Australian drug policy during this time was dominated by a range of adjustments to existing legislation that modified the definition of drug offences to make their conviction easier and their punishment harsher (Manderson 1993).

Adjustments to the legislation of drug offences also predictably translated into significant increases in the concentration of policing and law enforcement. During the 1970s, the Australian Bureau of Statistics recorded spikes in rates of drug offences in all jurisdictions around the country. In 1974–1975, NSW recorded 83.6 (per 100,000 population) drug offences, with Queensland recording 87.5 and 53.1 in Victoria: by 1977–1978 those rates had raised to 204.4 (NSW), 135.7 (Qld) and 99.7 (Vic), respectively (Wardlaw and Deane 1986). The authors of an Australian Institute of Criminology (AIC) report noted that these data are largely a "measure of police activity", and is thus limited in its ability to quantify apparent increases in drug use itself (Wardlaw and Deane 1986: 2). It is also worth noting that within the larger jurisdictions, such as NSW and Qld, offences related to the selling or supply of drugs consistently remained lower than 10% of all recorded drug offences. This reveals a formulaic targeting of user-level populations for drug law enforcement that mimicked the approach of the DEA.

It is useful to reflect on what this kind of policing reveals about the governance of Australian citizens at the time and its resonance with contemporary forms of drug-related law enforcement. The targeting of street-level drug use assumes that people who use drugs have the capacity to 'choose otherwise' and thus the threat of criminal charges is presented as a method to deter illicit consumption (Aitken et al. 2002; Cooper et al. 2005). Systems of law enforcement that target people who use drugs as a form of deterrence reduce choices about 'risky behavior' to a simple matter of rational calculation: comparisons to the neoliberal emphasis on the responsibilization of health practice (Petersen and Lupton 1996) are salient. This model tends to obscure social structures that produce the kind of marginalization present in the communities in which dependent drug use is most common (Meares 1997). The police targeting of individual drug consumers has also been critiqued for amplifying the 'risk environment' in which drug use occurs (Moore 2004). Despite its limitations and shortcomings, the policing of street-level drug use remains a significant component of contemporary law enforcement, particularly as it relates to injecting drug use (Aitken et al. 2002).

In Australia, the shadow of an international 'war on drugs' translated into accounts of a 'social problem' characterized by the 'deviance' of people who use drugs. Rather than directing the majority of policing resources to the health needs of people who use drugs, or to interrupt the manufacture and sale of drugs, the 1970s saw notable increases in police targeting of individual drug users. While the criminalizing imperative of this approach had popular support, sections of the community welfare and public health sectors began to emphasize the need to focus on better health and social outcomes.

Harm Minimization

Harm minimization policy and advocacy emerged out of a series of overlapping interests in politics, medicine and public health. In Australia, it was made possible because of the tragic circumstances that surrounded the daughter of a sitting Prime Minister. At a press conference in 1984, Bob Hawke revealed that his daughter was a "heroin addict". The announcement introduced unprecedented interest in and activity around Australian drug policy (McArthur 1999a). In April of the next year, the Prime Minister and the Premiers and Chief Ministers of all seven States and Territories gathered for a meeting in the nation's capital, Canberra. The meeting resulted in the creation of a new policy program to address drug use in Australia called the National Campaign Against Drug Abuse. The name of the policy was eventually changed to the less moralistic National Drug Strategy (NDS), but the fundamentals of a three-pronged approach to reduce the supply, demand and harm of drugs have remained unchanged (Lewis and MacPherson 2007). The new policy was significant because it adopted, what was termed a harm reduction component.

Given the context in which this new initiative was formed, harm minimization is often held up as a 'balanced approach' developed with "strong bipartisan political support" (Australian Government 2013). However, the new policy introduced in 1985 gave no definition for the harm reduction component, and it subsequently became exposed to the competing and conflicting agendas that comprise drug regulation: '"harm minimization" is that most unfortunate of beings—a term in search of a meaning' (Wodak and Saunders 1995). For years preceding its introduction, 'harm minimization' had been broadly applied to any policy measures that claimed to 'reduce harm' associated with drug use. This included prohibitionist and policing strategies, as well as public health and treatment programs. A clearer impression of the policy agenda can be located in the kinds of programs that have since become closely associated with a framework of harm minimization.

Joining a growing chorus of concern over the HIV/AIDs epidemic gripping many parts of the world, harm minimization proponents found a defining victory in the establishment of needle and syringe programs (NSP) in the late 1980s (Inciardi et al. 2009). NSPs provide sterile-injecting equipment to people who inject drugs so that they are discouraged from sharing needles that may carry blood-borne viruses. The spread of HIV in the 1980s was associated with the gay and injecting drug use populations of industrial nations (Blattner 1991). The introduction of NSP was born out of anxiety about the spread of HIV to other, less stigmatized, parts of the community. Its origins outside Australia are also most closely tied to the neoliberal health policies of the conservative Thatcher government in the UK (O'Hare 2007).

Since the 1980s, sections of public health have taken up a neoliberal philosophy that places emphasis on individual responsibility for health. Petersen and Lupton have described this trend as part of the emergence of what has been termed 'the new public health', which is 'at its core a moral enterprise' (1996: 174). As classic modernist institutions, medicine and epidemiology rely on the production of 'expert knowledge' about health and the ways of life that maximize health outcomes. Neoliberal health policy assumes that people have equal access to knowledge about health, unmitigated by circumstance or sociality, and that people therefore have the capacity to make 'healthy life choices'. As noted above, a similar philosophy informs policing practices that target street-based injecting drug use. As part of a philosophy about this kind of responsibilization of health care, Thatcher adopted a program of needle and syringe exchanges in the UK in 1986. With the support of medical and public health practitioners, Australia's first NSP was established in the same year, with a national network of programs implemented over the next few years (Wodak and Cooney 2005).

The precedent set by the introduction of NSP galvanized advocacy efforts around an alternative to prohibitionist policies. This provided many harm minimization advocates with a defining purpose that was distinct from the responsibilization of health endorsed by Thatcher. Harm minimization advocates emerged with a clear goal, to "prevent the baleful consequences of drug use without setting out to achieve this objective by interfering with drug consumption" (Wodak and Saunders 1995: 269). Proponents of prohibition constantly accuse this kind of harm minimization agenda of 'sending the wrong message', and implicitly endorsing illicit consumption. This is illustrative of an important philosophical distinction between prohibitionist policies that seek to address imagined future harms to society and harm minimization initiatives that address immediate harm to people who use drugs. There are, however, other policies that are presented under a harm minimization framework that demonstrate a blurrier model of reducing harm.

Since the 1980s, the use of opioid substitution treatment (OST) has also been largely framed as a harm minimization initiative. OST provides a stable prescription of a pharmaceutical opiate to medically maintain people who are dependent on opiates. The continued consumption and indeed prescription of a psychoactive drug are important in its subsequent integration into harm minimization frameworks. American researchers Dole and Nyswander are largely credited with establishing the medical viability of OST in a study using methadone. Dole and Nyswander reported marked shifts in the behavior of patients who received daily doses of methadone and argued that medically maintaining people who are drug dependent, even if it was for the rest of their lives, would serve to reduce morbidity, mortality, crime, and other associated social problems (Dole and Nyswander 1967).

Methadone was introduced to Australia in the experimental capacity of an opioid substitution drug in the early 1970s and has been used with varying popularity and success ever since (McArthur 1999b). High-dose formulations of buprenorphine for the treatment of dependence became available in Australia in the mid-2000s (Jenkinson et al. 2005). Buprenorphine–naloxone was introduced to Australia in 2006, largely in response to concerns that buprenorphine—and to a lesser extent methadone—was being diverted to illicit markets and injected (Larance et al. 2011).

Despite being presented under the humanitarian framework of harm minimization, critiques of the administration of OST have pointed to the constraints they place on clients. The status of OST as harm minimization is complicated by the fact that most prescribers and dispensers specify abstinence from heroin or other opiate injecting, among an array of other behavioral requirements, in order to stay on the program. Authors such as Bourgois (2000), Friedman and Alicea (2001), and Harris and McElrath (2012) even accuse US methadone programs of operating as a form of medical surveillance that chemically leashes clients, limiting their ability to fully participate in society. Australian researchers Fraser and Valentine provide a more nuanced account of methadone programs in Victoria and New South Wales by describing how they both reproduce and interrupt typical accounts of 'drug addiction' (Fraser and Valentine 2008).

While harm minimization was being defined throughout the 1980s, drug policy presented a highly conflicted account of prohibitionist (supply and demand reduction) and public health (harm reduction) philosophies. As a result, prohibitionist discourse itself began to adapt to compensate for the humanitarian concerns raised by those advocating harm minimization, though not necessarily to the benefit of people who use drugs. Throughout the 1980s, prohibition advocates in Australia began to frame their policy agenda as in defense of people "falling victim" to the criminal activities of "drug pushers" (Manderson 1993). Law enforcement also adjusted its rhetoric to focus on the traffic and sale of drugs. A new political discourse soon emerged that made an explicit distinction between 'users' and 'dealers'.

The user/dealer distinction became a political tool, lending the national policy of drug enforcement the appearance that it was operating in the interest of people who use drugs. Yet the practicalities of policing illicit drug markets left people who use drugs arguably even more exposed to law enforcement and the criminal justice system (Maher and Dixon 2001; Rowe 2005). The dichotomization of 'users' and 'dealers' ignores their obvious interconnectedness. Many people who use drugs regularly often also sell them to support their dependence (Maher 2000). In the policing of drugs, the two worlds thus become inseparable, because people who use drugs have obvious insight into the activities of those who sell them and are much easier to identify than 'dealers' and 'traffickers'. This led to a reinvigorated pursuit of people who use drugs, who were often intimidated into cooperation with the threat of criminal charges, and rarely presented with therapeutic options (Chambliss 1995).

As Australia moved into the 1990s and 2000s, tensions between advocacy efforts that centered on harm minimization and policy agendas that emphasized prohibition were becoming increasingly pronounced. Though the official harm reduction policy continued, and its support from specialist medical and public health domains remained, little was being done to implement a harm minimization agenda. In an effort to combat HIV transmission and related harms through less punitive measures, a range of user organizations were established. The Australian Injecting and Illicit Drug Users League (AIVL) began community health work in the late 1980s and became a fully incorporated association in 1992. Similar activist and community organizations were also formed at the state level, most notably with the NSW Users and AIDS Association (NUUA) in 1989. Leading into the twenty-first century, AIVL, NUUA and similar organizations began to establish momentum for advocacy of harm minimization.

However in November 1997, at the leadership of then Prime Minister John Howard, the new conservative government announced its drug strategy, openly introducing drug war rhetoric onto the national stage (Mendes 2007). Prime Minister Howard himself vetoed a bill that would have initiated a heroin trial in the ACT "despite years of multidisciplinary feasibility studies and the approval of a majority of the state, territory and federal police and health ministers" (Mendes 2007: 5). In light of rhetorical opposition at the Federal level, harm minimization became symbolic of an alternative to the prohibitionist policies that were failing many communities across Australia.

The late 1990s saw reports of a 'heroin drought' in Australia dominate media coverage of drug use (Poynting and Morgan 2007). A significant spike in heroin overdose deaths in inner-city suburbs of Sydney quickly followed. On January 31, 1999, The Sun-Herald published a photograph of what appeared to be a 15-year-old being injected with heroin by a staff member at an NSP in Carline Lane, Redfern. On the cusp a state election, the image and accompanying article sparked a political row over the effectiveness of the state's NSPs. Bob Carr's State Labor Government won reelection having promised the initiation of a Drug Summit, which eventually recommended, among other things, the establishment of a supervised injecting site. Despite some public opposition, Sydney's Medically Supervised Injecting Centre (MSIC), the first of its kind in the world, opened on a trial basis in May of 2001 (Freeman et al. 2005).

MSIC has become firmly identified as a harm minimization measure that seeks to reduce the harms associated with drugs without necessarily reducing drug use itself. Evaluations of the facility in 2003 and 2007 both provided compelling evidence that the MSIC was affordably achieving its goal to reduce many of the harms associated with drug use. The NSW government extended the trial basis of the facility following each successful evaluation (van Beek et al. 2004). After operating for nearly 10 years on a trial basis, the NSW government legislated the facility as a permanent fixture in 2010.

Conclusion

The histories discussed in this chapter reveal important societal changes that were variously responsible for and the consequence of shifting approaches to drugs. The medical profession has played a leading role in the regulation of analgesic and opiate consumption over the last century. Importantly, medicine has defined the socially constructed distinctions between the legal and therapeutic status of drugs. This has, however, contributed to the development of naïve discourse about 'good' and 'bad' drugs, 'benign' and 'addictive' consumption, and at times disguised the harms associated with legal medications and exaggerated the harms of illicit drugs (Manderson 1993). Medical discourse has also been used to legitimize increasingly punitive drug policy and policing practice, which in many cases produces harms of its own (Levine 2003). The historical influence of medicine is tied to political and professional interests that are often presented under the guise of scientific consensus.

The encroachment of consumer and neoliberal discourses informs a degree of contestation to medical and legal authorities in the field of drug regulation. The commercial and class interests that propelled neoliberal policies about the entrepreneurial capacity of the individual in the 'free market' form part of a trend toward self-regulation. Public health has at times borrowed from the neoliberal philosophy of individual responsibility for health (Petersen and Lupton 1996), most notably with the introduction of NSP in the UK and Australia (Zibbell 2004). Though harm minimization is more closely associated with activist movements and community organizations, its policies often involve a call to allow the individual the responsibility to regulate their own consumption of drugs.

Frameworks of medical and self-regulation of drugs in Australia have also been intimately tied to moral judgments about the people who are consuming them and the lives they lead. Opposition to Chinese migration and opium smoking emerged alongside objections to the apparent threat posed by the presence and 'sexual perversity' of the 'Chinaman' in Australia in the early twentieth century. The pathologization of over-the-counter analgesic use in Australia as a 'female problem' is illustrative of the way drug use and its regulation has been used as a form of social control. The historical influence of addiction in medical research has also produced moralized distinctions between different paths to drug dependence and the way they are policed in the shadow of a 'war on drugs'. These moral positions are juxtaposed with the unthreatening use of pharmaceuticals and alcohol, whose characterization as 'safe' was propelled by the implementation of the PBS and liberalization of alcohol legislation during the middle part of the twentieth century.

By taking a historical perspective, this chapter has demonstrated how transformations in Australian approaches to drug regulation have little to do with the scientific 'discovery' of the harmful properties of illicit drugs. Rather, forms of medical and self-regulation appear to intersect with the legal and moral histories that make up the political economy of drug consumption. These regulatory frameworks remain contested and fluid, presenting a series of tensions between medical authority, political influence, social change, commercial interests and neoliberal discourse. As a result, painkillers and analgesics emerge as intermediary objects that slip between the categories of legal and illegal, medical and non-medical, and moral and immoral, depending on the context of consumption. The histories of drug use discussed in the chapter provide a critical framework for understanding the way drug use is framed, both in research and as an issue of public policy.

References

Acker, C. J. (2002). *Creating the American Junkie: Addiction Research in the Classic Era of Narcotic Control.* Baltimore and London: Johns Hopkins University Press.

Aitken, C., Moore, D., Higgs, P., Kelsall, J., & Kerger, M. (2002). The Impact of a Police Crackdown on a Street Drug Scene: Evidence from the Street. *International Journal of Drug Policy, 13*(3), 193–202.

Australian Academy of Science. (2013). *Professor Priscilla Kincaid-Smith, Nephrologist.* Retrieved April 28, 2017, from https://www.science.org.

au/learning/general-audience/history/interviews-australian-scientists/professor-priscilla-kincaid-smith.

Australian Government. (2013). *National Drug Strategy*. Retrieved February 1, 2014, from http://www.nationaldrugstrategy.gov.au/.

Baer, W., & Maloney, W. (1997). Neoliberalism and Income Distribution in Latin America. *World Development, 25*(3), 311–327.

Biggs, A. (2002). *The Pharmaceutical Benefits Scheme—An Overview. E-Breifing—Social Policy Group*. Retrieved April 28, 2017, from http://www.aph.gov.au/About_Parliament/Parliamentary_Departments/Parliamentary_Library/Publications_Archive/archive/pbs.

Billington, B. P. (1960). The Australian Gastric Ulcer Change: Further Observations. *Medical Journal of Australia, 47*(2), 19–20.

Billington, B. P. (1963). The Australian Gastric Ulcer Change: Interstate Variations. *Australasian Annals of Medicine, 12,* 153–159.

Blattner, W. A. (1991). HIV Epidemiology: Past, Present, and Future. *The FASEB Journal, 5*(10), 2340–2348.

Blocker, J. S., Fahey, D. M., & Tyrrell, I. R. (2003). *Alcohol and Temperance in Modern History: An International Encyclopedia*. Santa Barbara, Denver, and Oxford, UK: Abc-Clio Incorporated.

Bourgois, P. (2000). Disciplining Addictions: The Bio-Politics of Methadone and Heroin in the United States. *Culture, Medicine, Psychiatry, 24*(2), 165–195.

Bourgois, P. (2002). Anthropology and Epidemiology on Drugs: The Challenges of Cross-Methodological and Theoretical Dialogue. *International Journal of Drug Policy, 13*(4), 259–269.

Brereton, D. (2000). The History and Politics of Prohibition. In G. Stokes, P. Chalk, & K. Gillen (Eds.), *Drugs and Democracy: In Search of New Directions*. Melbourne: Melbourne University Press.

Burnley, I. H. (1982). *Population, Society and Environment in Australia*. Melbourne: Shillington House.

Campbell, N. D. (2007). *Discovering Addiction: The Science and Politics of Substance Abuse Research*. Ann Arbor: University of Michigan Press.

Carney, T. (1981). The History of Australian Drug Laws: Commercialism to Confusion? *Monash University Law Review, 7*(3), 165–204.

Chambliss, W. J. (1995). Another Lost War: The Costs and Consequences of Drug Prohibition. *Social Justice, 22*(2), 101–124.

Commonwealth of Australia. (2013). *About the PBS*. Retrieved March 10, 2012, from http://www.pbs.gov.au/info/about-the-pbs.

Conrad, P., & Leiter, V. (2004). Medicalization, Markets and Consumers. *Journal of Health and Social Behaviour, 45,* 158–176.
Conrad, P., & Schneider, J. W. (1980). *Deviance and Medicalization: From Badness to Sickness.* Philadelphia: Temple University Press.
Cooper, H., Moore, L., Gruskin, S., & Krieger, N. (2005). The Impact of a Police Drug Crackdown on Drug Injectors' Ability to Practice Harm Reduction: A Qualitative Study. *Social Science and Medicine, 61*(3), 673–684.
Crawford, R. (1980). Healthism and the Medicalization of Everyday Life. *International Journal of Health Services, 10*(3), 365–388.
De Vogli, R. (2011). Neoliberal Globalisation and Health in a Time of Economic Crisis. *Social Theory & Health, 9*(4), 311–325.
Dole, V., & Nyswander, M. (1967). Heroin Addiction—A Metabolic Disease. *Archives of Internal Medicine, 120*(1), 19–24.
Dreisbach, R. H., & Pfeiffer, C. (1943). Caffeine Withdrawal Headache. *Journal of Laboratory Clinical Medicine, 28,* 1212–1219.
Duster, T. S. (1970). *The Legislation of Morality: Law, Drugs, and Moral Judgment.* New York: The Free Press.
Dyster, B., & Meredith, D. (1990). *Australia in the International Economy: In the Twentieth Century.* Cambridge: Cambridge University Press.
Fitzgerald, R., & Jordan, T. (2011). *Under the Influence: A History of Alcohol in Australia.* Sydney: HarperCollins.
Fraser, S., & Valentine, K. (2008). *Substance and Substitution: Methadone Subjects in Liberal Societies.* Basingstoke: Palgrave Macmillan.
Freeman, K., Jones, C. G., Weatherburn, D. J., Rutter, S., Spooner, C. J., & Donnelly, N. (2005). The Impact of the Sydney Medically Supervised Injecting Centre (MSIC) on Crime. *Drug and Alcohol Review, 24*(2), 173–184.
Freidson, E. (1988). *Profession of Medicine: A Study of the Sociology of Applied Knowledge.* Chicago and London: University of Chicago Press.
Friedman, J., & Alicea, M. (2001). *Surviving Heroin: Interviews with Women in Methadone Clinics.* Gainesville: University Press of Florida.
Gahlinger, P. (2004). *Illegal Drugs: A Complete Guide to Their History, Chemistry, Use, and Abuse.* New York: Plume Publications.
Galea, S., Ahern, J., & Vlahov, D. (2003). Contextual Determinants of Drug Use Risk Behavior: A Theoretical Framework. *Journal of Urban Health, 80(4*), iii50–iii58.

Gault, M. H., Rudwal, T. C., Engles, W. D., & Dossetor, J. B. (1968). Syndrome Associated with the Abuse of Analgesics. *Annals of Internal Medicine, 68*(4), 906–923.

Hamilton, M., Kellehear, A., & Rumbold, G. (1998). *Drug Use in Australia: A Harm Minimisation Approach*. Melbourne: Oxford University Press.

Harris, J., & McElrath, K. (2012). Methadone as Social Control: Institutionalized Stigma and the Prospect of Recovery. *Qualitative Health Research, 22*(6), 810–824.

Hartman, S. M. (1978). Prescriptions for Penelope. *Women's Studies, 5*(3), 223.

Harvey, D. (2005). *A Brief History of Neoliberalism*. Oxford: Oxford University Press.

Hennessey, E. (1992). 'Her Stand-by for Keeping Going' APC Use During the Boom Decades. *Journal of the Royal Historical Society of Queensland, 15*(5), 248–264.

Hennessey, E. (1993). *A Cup of Tea, a Bex, and a Good Lie Down*. Department of History & Politics, James Cook University of North Queensland.

Hogshire, J., & Alfvegren, S. (1999). *Pills-A-Go-Go: A Fiendish Investigation into Pill Marketing, Art, History and Consumption*. Venice, CA: Feral House.

Inciardi, J. A., Surratt, H. L., Cicero, T. J., & Beard, R. A. (2009). Prescription Opioid Abuse and Diversion in an Urban Community: The Results of an Ultrarapid Assessment. *Pain Medicine, 10*(3), 537–548.

Jackson, B. (1966). *White-Collar Party*. Atlantic, August 1966 Issue.

Jenkinson, R. A., Clark, N. C., Fry, C. L., & Dobbin, M. (2005). Buprenorphine Diversion and Injection in Melbourne, Australia: An Emerging Issue? *Addiction, 100*, 197–205.

Keane, H., & Hamill, K. (2010). Variations in Addiction: The Molecular and the Molar in Neuroscience and Pain Medicine. *BioSocieties, 5*(1), 52–69.

Kincain-Smith, P. (1969). Analgesic Nephropathy: A Common Form of Renal Disease in Australia. *Medical Journal of Australia, 2*, 1131–1135.

Kolb, L. (1962). *Drug Addiction: A Medical Problem*. Springfield, IL: Thomas Books.

Lake, M., & Reynolds, H. (2008). *Drawing the Global Colour Line: White Men's Countries and the International Challenge of Racial Equality*. Melbourne, VIC: Cambridge University Press.

Larance, B., Degenhardt, L., Lintzeris, N., Winstock, A., & Mattick, R. (2011). Definitions Related to the Use of Pharmaceutical Opioids: Extramedical Use, Diversion, Non-Adherence and Aberrant Medication-Related Behaviours. *Drug and Alcohol Review, 30*(3), 236–245.

Leonard, K. E. (2002). Alcohol's Role in Domestic Violence: A Contributing Cause or an Excuse? *Acta Psychiatrica Scandinavica, 106*(s412), 9–14.
Levine, H. G. (1978). The Discovery of Addiction: Changing Conceptions of Habitual Drunkenness in America. *Journal of Studies on Alcohol, 39*(1), 143–174.
Levine, H. G. (1993). Temperance Cultures: Alcohol as a Problem in Nordic and English-Speaking Cultures. In M. Lader, E. Griffith, & D. C. Colin (Eds.), *The Nature of Alcohol and Drug Related Problems*. Oxford: Oxford University Press.
Levine, H. G. (2003). Global Drug Prohibition: Its Uses and Crises. *International Journal of Drug Policy, 14*(2), 145–153.
Lewis, M. J., & MacPherson, K. L. (2007). *Public Health in Australia from the Nineteenth to the Twenty-First Century Public Health in Asia and the Pacific: Historical and Comparative Perspectives*. Abingdon: Taylor & Francis.
Lupton, G. M., & Najman, J. M. (1995). *Sociology of Health and Illness: Australian Readings*. Melbourne: Paul & Company Pub Consortium.
Maher, L. (2000). *Sexed Work: Gender, Race and Resistance in a Brooklyn Drug Market*. Oxford: Oxford University Press.
Maher, L., & Dixon, D. (2001). Cost of Crackdowns: Policing Cabramatta's Heroin Market. *Current Issues in Criminal Justice, 13*(1), 5–22.
Manderson, D. (1988). The First Loss of Freedom: Early Opium Laws in Australia. *Drug and Alcohol Review, 7*(4), 439–453.
Manderson, D. (1993). *From Mr Sin to Mr Big: A History of Australian Drug Laws*. Melbourne: Oxford University Press.
Manderson, D. (1995). The Semiotics of the Title: A Comparative and Historical Analysis of Drug Legislation. *Law, Text, Culture, 2,* 160–178.
Manderson, D. (1999). Symbolism and Racism in Drug History and Policy. *Drug and Alcohol Review, 18*(2), 179–186.
Manderson, D. (2005). Possessed: Drug Policy, Witchcraft and Belief. *Cultural Studies, 19*(1), 36–63.
McArthur, M. (1999a). Pushing the Drug Debate: The Media's Role in Policy Reform. *Australian Journal of Social Issues, 34*(2), 149–165.
McArthur, M. (1999b). *A History of Methadone Treatment in Australia: The Influence of Social Control Arguments in Its Development*. Paper Presented at the History of Crime, Policing and Punishment Conference, Canberra.
Meares, T. L. (1997). Social Organization and Drug Law Enforcement. *American Criminal Law Review, 35,* 191.

Mendes, P. (2007). Fighting the Drugs War: The Role of Prohibitionist Groups in Australian Illicit Drugs Policy. *Practice Reflections, 2*(1), 3–16.

Miles, A. (1953). Pills: Are They a Help or a Menace? *Baltimore Afro-American*. Retrieved October 25, from http://news.google.com/newspapers?nid=2205&dat=19551025&id=_OYlAAAAIBAJ&sjid=cfUFAAAAIBAJ&pg=2329,1952799.

Miller, S. (2009). *Chapter Four: Context of the National Straterg*y (NDS Final Report Vol. 1). Department of Health and Aging.

Moore, D. (2004). Governing Street-Based Injecting Drug Users: A Critique of Heroin Overdose Prevention in Australia. *Social Science and Medicine, 59*(7), 1547–1557.

Murray, R. (1980). Minor Analgesic Abuse: The Slow Recognition of a Public Health Problem. *British Journal of Addiction, 75*(1), 9–17.

Nadesan, M. H. (2008). *Governmentality, Biopower, and Everyday Life*. New York: Routledge.

Navarro, V. (2007). *Neoliberalism, Globalization, and Inequalities: Consequences for Health and Quality of Life*. Amityville: Baywood Publishing.

O'Hare, P. (2007). Merseyside, the First Harm Reduction Conferences, and the Early History of Harm Reduction. *International Journal of Drug Policy, 18*(2), 141–144.

Petersen, A., & Lupton, D. (1996). *The New Public Health: Health and Self in the Age of Risk*. London: Sage.

Poynting, S., & Morgan, G. (2007). *Outrageous!: Moral Panics in Australia*. Hobart: Australian Clearinghouse for Youth Studies.

Phillips, W. (1980). 'Six O'Clock Swill': The Introduction of Early Closing of Hotel Bars in Australia. *Historical Studies, 19*(75), 250–266.

Punch, M. (2005). Problem Drug Use and the Political Economy of Urban Restructuring: Heroin. *Class and Governance in Dublin. Antipode, 37*(4), 754–774.

Purdie, N., Dudgeon, P., & Walker, R. (2010). *Working Together: Aboriginal and Torres Strait Islander Mental Health and Wellbeing Principles and Practice*. Department of Health and Aging: Australian Government.

Race, K. (2005). Recreational States: Drugs and the Sovereignty of Consumption [Special Issue on Biopolitics]. *Culture Machine, 7*.

Ray, O. S. (1978). *Drugs, Society, and Human Behavior*. St. Louis: C.V. Mosby Co.

Reiner, R. (2012). What's Left? The Prospects for Social Democratic Criminology. *Crime, Media, Culture, 8*(2), 135–150.

Rolfe, J. L. (1989). *Legal Alternatives and Consequences. Historical Paper: Legislative Developments*. Melbourne: Drug Research & Rehabilitation Fund.

Room, R. (2005). Stigma, Social Inequality and Alcohol and Drug Use. *Drug and Alcohol Review, 24*(2), 143–155.

Room, R. (2010). The Long Reaction Against the Wowser: The Prehistory of Alcohol Deregulation in Australia. *Health Sociology Review, 19*(2), 151–163.

Rowe, J. (2005). From Deviant to Disenfranchised: The Evolution of Drug Users in AJSI. *Australian Journal of Social Issues, 40*(1), 107–123.

Shelley, J. H. (1967). Phenacetin Through the Looking Glass. *Clinical Pharmacology and Therapeutics, 8*(3), 427–471.

Singer, M. (2008). Drugs and Development: The Global Impact of Drug Use and Trafficking on Social and Economic Development. *International Journal of Drug Policy, 19*(6), 467–478.

Stelle, T. W., Gyory, A. Z., & Edwards, K. D. G. (1969). Renal Function in Analgesic Nephropathy. *British Medical Journal, 2*, 213–216.

Stewart, H. H. (1978). Analgesic Abuse and Renal Failure in Australasia. *Kidney International, 13*, 72–78.

Sulkunen, P., & Warpenius, K. (2000). Reforming the Self and the Other: The Temperance Movement and the Duality of Modern Subjectivity. *Critical Public Health, 10*(4), 423–438.

Sydney City & Suburban Sewage and Health Board. (1875–1876). *Eleventh Progress Report in NSW Legislative Assembly, Votes and Proceedings, 5*, 535–661.

United Nations Office on Drugs and Crime. (2008). *Drug Policy and Results in Australia October 2008*.

van Beek, I., Kimber, J., Dakin, A., & Gilmour, S. (2004). The Sydney Medically Supervised Injecting Centre: Reducing Harm Associated with Heroin Overdose. *Critical Public Health, 14*(4), 391–406.

Wardlaw, G., & Deane, H. (1986). *Uses and Abuses of Drug Law Enforcement Statistics*. Australian Institute of Criminology, Trends and Issues in Crime and Criminal Justice.

Willis, E. (1989). *Medical Dominance: The Division of Labour in Australian Health Care*. Sydney: Allen & Unwin.

Wilkinson, R. G., & Marmot, G. (2003). *Social Determinants of Health: The Solid Facts*. World Health Organization, Regional Office for Europe.

Wodak, A., & Cooney, A. (2005). Effectiveness of Sterile Needle and Syringe Programmes. *International Journal of Drug Policy, 16*(1), 31–44.

Wodak, A., & Owens, R. (1996). *Drug Prohibition: A Call for Change*. Sydney: UNSW Press.

Wodak, A., & Saunders, B. (1995). Harm Reduction Means What I Choose It to Mean. *Drug and Alcohol Review, 14*(3), 269–271.

Young, J. (2011). Moral Panics and the Transgressive Other. *Crime, Media, Culture, 7*(3), 245–258.

Zibbell, J. E. (2004). Can the Lunatics Actually Take Over the Asylum?: Reconfiguring Subjectivity and Neo-Liberal Governance in Contemporary British Drug Treatment Policy. *International Journal of Drug Policy, 15*(1), 56–65.

Zinberg, N. E. (1986). *Drug, Set, and Setting: The Basis for Controlled Intoxicant Use*. New Haven: Yale University Press.

3

'Discovering' Non-Medical (Ab)Use: The Meaning and Measurement of Non-Medical Consumption

A growing body of research has adopted a discourse of 'abuse' to describe the non-medical consumption of pharmaceutical pain medications. In a manner comparable with their role in distinguishing between 'licit' and 'illicit' opiates, the medical profession has played a key role in extending a discourse of abuse to include the consumption of analgesic medications in unauthorized ways. Where the previous chapter identified the sociohistorical context under which pain medications became the antithesis of 'street drugs', this chapter outlines changes in research discourse about pain medications and their capacity to be 'misused'. The medical literature now commonly presents non-medical 'painkiller abuse' as a scientific 'discovery' about an apparently new and emerging drug problem.

This chapter performs two central tasks through a critical review of the available literature: first, it examines the conceptual frameworks upon which this growing body of primarily US literature is based; second, it addresses the way these frameworks inform Australian research and commentary about non-medical (ab)use. The chapter begins with a critical evaluation of the influential definition of the (US) Substance Abuse and Mental Health Services Administration (SAMHSA) of the

G. C. Dertadian, *A Fine Line*,
https://doi.org/10.1007/978-981-13-1975-4_3

US Department of Health and Human Services. It then discusses the terminology used in the dissemination of epidemiological research and addresses the way clinical literature produces practices of non-medical consumption within pathologizing frameworks.

Much North American research is underpinned by an emphasis on medical authority and a tendency toward pathologization, which in turn informs Australian research and policy responses to the non-medical use of painkillers. The remainder of the chapter thus focuses specifically on the Australian context. Assessment of Australian literature starts with a review of national data collection and its limitations. This includes an analysis of questions about non-medical use in the Illicit Drug Reporting System (IDRS), the Drug Use Monitoring in Australia (DUMA) project and the National Drug Strategy Household Survey (NDSHS). Smaller studies, and institutional and government responses are also considered. In surveying the research literature, this chapter provides a critical assessment of the kind of knowledge being produced about non-medical use through such research.

Defining the Practice

Most research into non-medical consumption uses the definition of the SAMHSA of the US Department of Health and Human Services. As advised by the SAMHSA "non-medical use" is usually thought to refer to "the use of a prescription drug when 'it was not prescribed for you', or that was taken 'only for the experience or feeling it cause[s]'" (Sees et al. 2005). This definition articulates two broad categories of concern related to non-adherent medication consumption, based on (a) prescription as the only legitimate method of acquisition and (b) medically defined benefit as the only legitimate motive for consumption. These concerns are integrated throughout the research literature and are often used to infer dysfunction and criminality. This section will provide a brief assessment of the SAMHSA definition before elaborating on the impacts that definitional problems can have on the field of substance abuse prevention and treatment.

Beginning with the first concern, it is significant to note that the SAMHSA definition relates directly to prescription medications and makes no reference to over-the-counter medications. This is despite the fact that discourses of pharmaceutical (ab)use include apparent overuse of over-the-counter medications with sometimes serious health implications. However, the SAMHSA definition binds 'legitimate medical use' to 'ownership' of a specific prescription. The therapeutic action of a particular medical treatment is therefore irrelevant to this definition of abuse. Under the SAMHSA definition, use of the same medicine, for the same medical purpose, may well be rendered non-medical if it is acquired through a prescription addressed to a friend or family member. Here the actual effect of consumption becomes irrelevant to the definition, which is focused on the possible willful deceit of medical practitioners by patients or the use of prescriptions for purposes other than those intended by the practitioner.

A 2005 study utilizing the SAMHSA definition acknowledges how the limitations of this first criterion may produce a problematic reading of survey results:

> [a] positive answer to the specific survey question could mean that the respondent had... taken one dose of a specific pain reliever to treat pain, although the medication was not prescribed for that particular pain problem. While such use is clearly 'non-medical', it does not meet established criteria for 'abuse'. (Sees et al. 2005: 22)

The first criterion of the SAMHSA definition implies that 'legitimate' consumption is bound to an interaction within the medical clinic, between prescriber and patient. This kind of approach discounts any consideration of what might be happening in the life of the medication user outside the medical clinic. What if a patient's pain suddenly flares up when they are not in the presence of a doctor? Should they refuse a dose of their friend's pain medication simply because it was not prescribed to them? These kinds of considerations are left out of the SAMHSA definition and, as we shall see in the rest of the chapter, can be misleadingly implicated in discourses of dysfunction and crime.

The second dimension of the SAMHSA definition of non-medical consumption is focused on use for the sole purpose of the 'experience' or 'feeling' of the medication. This criterion is somewhat unique in terms of its influence in epidemiological research, which, as noted in the Chapter 1, has long neglected the role of pleasure in drug use (Moore 2008; Treloar and Holt 2006). Despite this emphasis on 'experience' and 'feeling', the epidemiological literature still tends to deal with pleasure-seeking as a criterion for non-medical use, rather than as a motivator for use. Chronic pain research challenges this delegitimization of drug consumption for 'subjective' reasons such as experience or feeling. Concerns about the under treatment of pain (Passik and Kirsh 2004), a worsening of the patient's condition (Littlejohn et al. 2004), or anxiety about the treatment of chronic pain (Kirsh et al. 2007), have all raised important questions about positioning the 'experience' or 'feeling' of painkiller use as problematic.

Chronic pain research has demonstrated that many patients actively seek the drug in question precisely for the experience or feeling that it causes (Kwon et al. 2014). Indeed, the experience or feeling of the drug is what acts as therapeutic and allows for the patient to live unburdened by crippling chronic pain, depression or anxiety. The next chapter will elaborate further on the significance of pain medicine, but for now it is relevant to note that, for patients with persistent pain problems, enjoying the relief that their medications provide may be entirely expected. How the SAMHSA distinguishes between 'experience' of the drug as recreational and as therapeutic is thus unclear. Moreover, there is little evidence that the recreational and therapeutic 'feeling' of drug consumption can in fact be separated so neatly. The blurred distinction between recreational release and therapeutic analgesia is a strong theme that emerges in interview in this study and will be dealt with in Part II of the book.

A final observation about the SAMHSA definition is that it attempts to produce generic criteria for 'legitimate medical use' and 'illegitimate non-medical abuse'. As was noted in the previous chapter, a substance's status as medication is closely tied to medical narratives about its therapeutic value within a treatment program. All pharmaceuticals have their own patent regulations under professional guidelines, and recommendations for the medical use of analgesics will differ from those of other medications. Generic guidelines about medical verses non-medical consumption seem to relate much more to medical authority than to therapeutic practice. Given the limitations described here, the SAMHSA definition presents a series of problems when used as an indicator for problematic 'abuse'.

Terminology in the Field

Following from the SAMHSA definition, terminology about non-medical use usually relates to either modes of acquisition or motives for consumption. In clinical discourse, there are multiple terms used to describe practices of non-medical use. A significant background to the terminology used in the literature is the way medical and scientific accounts describe 'abuse' of drugs generally. Part of the reason why attention has come to the term 'abuse' is because medical and scientific communities have sought to differentiate between the medically appropriate use of opiates and the medically unauthorized 'abuse' of the same substances. In a series of influential articles published by Nora Volkow, the director of the National Institute on Drug Abuse (NIDA), it is argued that, when 'substances of abuse' are not used to address a medical condition, this can result in "decreased dopamine function in addicted subjects [which] results in decreased sensitivity to non-drug-related stimuli (including natural reinforcers) and disrupts frontal inhibition, both of which contribute to compulsive drug intake and impaired inhibitory control" (Volkow et al. 2004: 557). This argument is extended to a description of analgesic abuse specifically, and a case is made for the monitoring and surveillance of young people who consume opiates based on the notion that their 'abuse' places them at risk of addiction (Compton and Volkow 2006a, b).

While use of the term 'abuse' provides an important backdrop to the way terms in the field are deployed, there are a wide range of terms used in the literature that need to be canvassed. Studies investigating the use of medications prescribed to someone other than the consumer refer to 'diversion' (Vivian et al. 2005), 'non-adherence'

(Arria et al. 2011), 'misuse' (Kelly and Parsons 2007) and 'abuse' (Catalano 2009). Research investigating the apparent misuse of pharmaceuticals for the 'experience' or 'feeling' they cause include terms such as 'harmful use' (World Health Organization 2013), 'dependent use' (Davey et al. 1995) or 'aberrant medication-related behavior' (Webster and Webster 2005). Though each term is purposefully defined in each study, their use is often inconsistent and even interchangeable. This section discusses the terminology of non-medical use and the role this vocabulary plays in establishing pharmaceutical 'abuse' as a coherent field of study.

Terminology related to the acquisition of pharmaceuticals deals specifically with how to categorize the way people who use medications non-medically gain access to them. The term 'doctor shopping' is used to describe the behavior of patients who consult "several prescribers during the same period and obtaining overlapping prescription orders from these different prescribers" (Pradel et al. 2010: 612). A report from the Victorian Drugs and Crime Prevention Committee goes as far as exploring the "possibility of a criminal law for 'doctor shopping'" (2007: 16). Doctor shopping is often spoken about as a form of what is termed 'diversion'. While some studies include non-medical consumption as part of the definition of diversion, most restrict use of the term to the supply of pharmaceuticals to 'illicit drug markets' (Ritter and Natale 2005). According to a report from NDARC, '"diversion" describes the unsanctioned supply of regulated pharmaceuticals from legal sources to the illicit drug market, or to a user for whom the drugs were not intended' (Degenhardt et al. 2007: viii).

Attempts to measure the diversion of pharmaceuticals into illicit markets may, however, overrepresent its role in practices of non-medical consumption because it conflates intention to on-sell drugs for profit with informal medication sharing. While respondents in studies of non-medical use consistently report family and friends as the most common source of access to medications, there is little discussion of practices of sharing. What references there are to acquiring medications from family and friends condemn them as 'illicit' or as a form of 'diversion' (Inciardi et al. 2009). The impact of people who take leftover medications or share them with family and friends on the resulting data is almost entirely ignored in the epidemiological literature.

A lack of attention to the social and cultural elements of networks of sharing reinforces discourses of 'abuse' and 'illegality'. Studies with a greater focus on the social and cultural aspects of drug use can provide some important insights here. In a qualitative study of methadone services in Victoria and New South Wales, Fraser and Valentine note how sharing medications can represent a practice of care (2008: 136). The authors observe that access to a steady supply of a medically prescribed opiate is precious, and that despite reducing their own supply and the risk of having it cut off entirely, clients often share their methadone with intimate partners and friends who do not have access to a treatment program. As distinct from clinical guidelines which condemn the sharing of methadone, interpretations of interview data with service providers, policy makers and clients reveal, what the authors refer to as the "alternative treatment identity" of "the lay carer" (Fraser and Valentine 2008: 136). The lay carer is one example of the kinds of alternative modes of understanding medication sharing that social and cultural approaches can bring to the study of non-medical use.

Terminology related to the motivation for consumption is framed more clearly around the authority of the medical practitioner. Medical perspectives tend to categorize consumption as either compliant to medical instruction or not. Investment in medical authority is most clearly framed through use of terms that specify deviation from direct medical instruction, like 'non-compliance' and 'non-adherence' (Fischer et al. 2010). Use of the terms non-compliance and non-adherence places the medical professional and the patient in a power relationship of clear dominance and subordination. Practitioners in the field of (drug) dependence treatment also utilize this kind of framework through reporting on the 'misuse' of OST such as methadone (Winstock and Lea 2010). A conservative approach to the adherence to medical instruction is often articulated as essential to the effective delivery of these kinds of drug treatment services.

There are also important ways in which medical authority is embedded in the definition of terms that relate to health outcomes. As defined by a NDARC report, the term 'harmful use' refers to "a pattern of drug use that is causing negative impacts upon health and may have negative social consequences" (Degenhardt et al. 2007: viii). The report does not define what it means by harmful 'impacts on health'. The term 'harmful use' is, however, most often used when referring to injecting drug use and HIV and other disease transmission. It is telling that 'harmful use' comes to describe injecting drugs use and HIV transmission in this literature, because both are marked by histories of highly moralized medical discourse (Dyson 1992; Rhodes et al. 2005).

There are also important moral connotations that apply to the identification of and attempts to calculate 'negative social consequences', especially when presented as an indication of health. What constitutes a negative social consequence varies considerably according to which social group one is referring to. A comparison to the criteria of 'social impairment' for the psychological diagnosis of 'substance use disorder' (SUD) is salient. Fraser and colleagues have argued that clinical reference to the 'social' often involves:

> a hierarchical ranking of pleasures, in which family life and wholesome pursuits (assumed to be accessible and appealing to all) are placed above solitary consumption or the wrong sort of friends. (Fraser et al. 2014: 42)

These are assumptions about socially and culturally specific contexts that are far from the goals of objective clinical discovery. Use of 'social harm' in epidemiological research also conflates the harms of criminalization with the harms of drug use. Terms such as 'harmful use' potentially ignore the social complexity of drug use in favor of a privileging of medical authority, and its apparent ability to determine what kinds of sociality are appropriate. As is also clear in the literature about injecting drug use and HIV transmission, non-adherence is often thought of as unsanctioned and consequently can come to be understood as a form of morally contentious or even criminal behavior.

A focus on doctor shopping and diversion, non-adherence and its apparent harms are also inadequate for any serious discussion of the way over-the-counter medications are consumed. It is not a crime, nor necessarily medically negligent to purchase over-the-counter medications and offer them to family members and friends. Moreover, very little scrutiny is expected of the consumption of over-the-counter medications once they have been purchased. For instance, it is common for a workplace to have a communal medicine cabinet, likely to be comprised of over-the-counter medications.

In a chapter of *The Drug Effect* (2011), Keane draws on the work of Rose to observe how, through exposure to the biotechnological advances of the past fifty years, the modern citizen operates in "biological styles of thought" (Keane 2011: 117). The chapter articulates how working environments increasingly position 'underperformance' as the product of sleep deprivation and attention deficit hyperactivity disorder (ADHD), and thus, it is often medicated. Keane notes how this process forms part of 'twenty-first-century styles of medical thought [that] move beyond a concern with health and disease to the goal of optimisation' (Keane 2011: 107). While Keane discusses medications prescribed for sleep deprivation and ADHD, her work provides important frameworks for addressing the use of over-the-counter medications for the goal of productivity. It is unclear how the use of over-the-counter medications for productivity would be considered under the SAMHSA definition of non-medical use and the terminology that has accompanied it.

Framing 'legitimate' consumption around compliance also ignores developments in aspects of the health and medical perspective over the last fifty years. The emergence of the patient's rights movement and influential neoliberal health policies that encourage self-care contribute to the way people consume their medications. The term 'extra-medical use' is perhaps the most interesting in this respect. Extra-medical use most often refers to consumption 'without a prescription, but does not exclude the possibility that the user may have medically driven reasons for using the drug' (Degenhardt et al. 2007: viii). This term helps to ameliorate some of the problems associated with determining that consumption of a drug for its 'experience' or 'feeling' is automatically entirely problematic. This term recognizes that patients may determine their own health problem and are capable of (self)medicating with potentially therapeutic effect. Use of the term is, however, often limited to the pain medicine literature.

Research on non-medical use utilizes a range of terms that are primarily based on the criteria set out in the SAMHSA definition. Terminology relating to the 'illicit' acquisition of pharmaceuticals often conflates informal medication sharing with intention to profit from the on-selling of medications. Terms used to describe reasons other than medically defined benefit for consumption inscribe unrealistic distinctions between therapeutic outcome and pleasurable experience. The terminology described in this section informs much of how research on non-medical (ab)use is collected and disseminated. There is, however, another significant term, 'addiction', which is worth canvassing in detail for its influence on research about non-medical consumption.

'Addiction' and the DSM-5

'Addiction' is a common concern of medical and epidemiological research about painkiller consumption. Clinical literature about non-medical use almost exclusively adopts a biomedical model of addiction based on the diagnostic criteria set out in the American Psychiatric Association's (APA) Diagnostic and Statistical Manual of Mental Disorders (DSM). There are, however, important debates about the biomedical and clinical definition of addiction that inform the criteria set out by the DSM, much of which is illustrated by changes implemented in the manual's latest incarnation, DSM-5.

Released in May 2013 the latest version of the DSM introduces significant changes to the diagnostic criteria of substance-related disorders that have been hotly debated within the psychiatric and psychological communities (Keane et al. 2011). The authors of the new manual emphasize that changes to individual disorders have been adopted in order to bring them in line with current research, and to ensure that the diagnostic criteria identify disorders with distinct underlying pathologies. Despite explanations about the importance of each disorder in the manual having a discrete neurobiological pathology, such considerations rarely form part of the diagnostic process outlined in the DSM-5 classification of 'addiction'.

The DSM-5 collapses its predecessor's categories of 'substance use' and 'substance dependence' onto a continuum of what is referred to as SUD. The criteria for SUD are also accompanied by clinical descriptions that refine the diagnostic process for individual substances. The manual therefore separates the use of individual substances into distinct disorders, such as 'cocaine use disorder', 'alcohol use disorder' and 'opiate use disorder'. Despite presenting the use of individual substances as discrete categories of disorder, the overarching diagnostic criteria for SUD are the same across all substances listed in the manual.

Subjective evaluation and reported behavior remain central to, what the DSM-5 now terms 'substance-related and addictive disorders'. The diagnosis of SUD requires the observed or reported presence of at least two of the eleven available criteria. Much of this criterion relies on highly subjective observations about perceptions of 'impaired control', 'social impairment' and 'risky use', with only two relating to the 'pharmacology' of tolerance and withdrawal (APA 2013). Fraser and colleagues have noted that:

> SUD assembles diverse elements such as harms, risk, misuse of time, loss of self-control, pathological desire and biological disturbance into the condition of addiction and locates it in within the individual. However, the identification and evaluation of harm is not an objective or technical exercise as it involves judgements about what a meaningful and productive life looks like. (2014: 44)

These kinds of subjective judgements also extend to the prioritization of medical authority in aspects of the SUD diagnosis. For instance, in the DSM-5 tolerance and withdrawal are no longer required for a diagnosis of SUD and their presence is instructed to be excluded if the patient is using opiates under the supervision of a medical practitioner.

A reduction in the centrality of tolerance and withdrawal from the DSM-5 diagnosis is closely tied to the rise of pain medicine. Pain medicine literature insists that pain patients have been stigmatized because 'drug dependence' (tolerance and withdrawal) has been unnecessarily conflated with 'drug addiction'. Partly because of the interests of the specialty of pain medicine, the authority of the medical practitioner can be used to discount the only verifiable link to the neurological processes involved in the diagnosis of SUD. This effectively renders tolerance and withdrawal irrelevant to the SUD diagnosis when a patient's opiate use is being supervised by a medical practitioner:

> The symptoms of dependence, withdrawal and tolerance, which used to be the markers of genuine addiction, have become polysemic signifiers whose meaning is dependent on the absence or presence of medical supervision. Medical authority renders them expected side effects of treatment, while outside the clinical space, when combined with certain social realities, they become signs of compulsive and disordered desire. (Fraser et al. 2014: 48)

While the DSM-5 presents a clinical consensus surrounding a set of observable 'addictive' behaviors, the diagnostic process it sets out seems to have little to do with the notion of 'drug addiction' as a disease entity, located in the neurobiology of people who use drugs.

Despite the limited capacity for the DSM-5 diagnosis to identify the neurological components of 'addiction', research that utilizes its criteria often assumes the presence of a biomedical disease. This has important implications on the dissemination of research about people who use opiates. The potential for survey results about subjective categories of behavior to be transformed into indicators of disease requires close scrutiny.

Psychological Literature

In clinical research, there are a series of psychological issues that are often correlated with non-medical use. Statistical and survey data reveal significant correlations between non-medical consumption with the 'abuse' of psychoactive substances and a range of psychological disorders. The definitions used in clinical studies most often refer to DSM criteria for a range of psychological conditions, though a significant proportion of the available research is based on the manual's previous incarnation, DSM-IV-TR. Studies that use DSM criteria often reproduce the presumption of disease that operates in references to addiction, conflating a range of psychological disorders. For instance, in a 2008 study on the non-medical use of prescription opiates, the authors make the following observation:

> We have found a prevalence of past-year non-medical use of prescription opioids of 4.5% in a survey of... approximately 10 million people. Such use represents misuse of a controlled medication and raises concern of self-medication, illicit drug use, medication non-adherence, overdose and, of special concern, the potential transition to a substance use disorder. (Becker et al. 2008: 41)

In this study, "[opiate] abuse and dependence were collapsed into one category since these conditions are clinically similar" (Becker et al. 2008: 40). Psychological concern about 'illicit substance use' and non-medical use are often conflated in the literature, and terms such as 'abuse' and 'dependence' are commonly regarded as similar enough not to differentiate in the dissemination of results.

The distinction between 'abuse' and 'dependence' is largely unclear in clinical literature, and the terms are often applied to the same behavior. One study might consider non-medical use with the observation that 'persons are classified with "abuse" of a particular substance only if they are not 'dependent' on that substance' (Sees et al. 2005), another collapses the two altogether (Becker et al. 2008), and a third will declare both to be "illicit use" (Vivian et al. 2005). It is clear from observations such as this that the field is characterized by inconsistency and that this results in the perception that non-medical use will inevitably lead to abusive/dependent behaviors. Inconsistency in the terminology is highly problematic when considering that most studies rely on the definition of non-medical use provided by the SAMHSA to establish a link between consumption and disorder.

'Abuse' of and dependence on medications are not only thought of as psychological disorders in and of themselves, they are often also presented as symptomatic of other forms of psychological dysfunction. Clinical anxiety in particular has been associated with non-medical use (Vivian et al. 2005). Again, most studies refer to the DSM criteria for establishing the presence of symptoms of anxiety, and the literature refers to strong "associations between lifetime anxiety and mood disorders" (Becker et al. 2008). One study's definition of those disorders states that:

> Generalised anxiety symptoms are defined as worrying a lot more than most people about everyday problems or being a lot more nervous or anxious than most people for half of the past year or more. (Becker et al. 2008)

What is absent from this definition is any consideration that anxiety may be an inevitable and indeed expected response to contextual circumstances or lived experiences. Under the DSM's definition, the material realities of the everyday circumstances that affect people who use medications are rendered substantially irrelevant. The assumption is that if study respondents demonstrate symptoms of an anxiety disorder, they confirm clinical observations about connections between non-medical use (or substance use more generally) and psychological dysfunction. The potentially confounding influence of additional factors (for example, chronic pain or a stressful life situation) that may be producing anxiety and act as motivators for non-medical use is ignored.

It is important to recognize that affective responses, like anxiety, are not simply biologically produced, but are also socially and culturally produced. This point will be elaborated on in the next chapter, by describing how the conditions of late-modern society are associated with feelings of insecurity, uncertainty and anxiety. The attribution of psychological dysfunction to presentations of anxious behavior and subsequent attempts to pathologize and then medicate anxiety, overlooks the arguably widespread social, economic and political antecedents to anxiety.

The context in which people consume their medications is absent from much of the psychological literature produced by North American research. This presents a series of problems with the resulting data, including problematic conflations of medication 'use', 'abuse' and 'dependence'. This leaves the impression that any form of non-medical consumption is potentially pathological. Survey results that may be capturing informal medication sharing and the pleasurable aspects of pain relief are subsequently disseminated as indicators of levels of psychological disorder. Similarly, the literature's discussion of anxiety presents decontextualized accounts of non-medical consumption that are presented as symptomatic of psychological dysfunction. These pathologizing processes have established an overly mechanical and simplified relationship between reports of anxiousness and psychological illness.

People Who Inject Drugs and the IDRS

Research specific to the Australian context is less extensive and tends to focus on people with established patterns of drug use. Most Australian data are collected as part of broader studies on alcohol and other drugs (AOD). A group of researchers based primarily at the National Drug and Alcohol Research Centre (NDARC) have sought greater consistency of terminology for research on non-medical use, with a 2007 report noting that "'misuse', 'non-medical use' and 'extra-medical use' are often used interchangeably in practice" (Degenhardt et al. 2007: viii). A 2011 review of the available literature advocates for a narrowing of the terms used in research contexts to minimize the ambiguities that can result from the inconsistent application of terms (Larance et al. 2011). Larance and colleagues recommend that consistent terminology will produce less problematic results and allow for a broader application across multiple disciplines. It is significant to note here that attempts to consolidate the field in this way are illustrative of a prevailing abuse/illicit understanding of practices of non-medical consumption in the Australian research context.

Two annual national projects and one tri-annual national study on drug use have introduced questions about non-medical use, and these studies make up most Australian data on the topic. This section will focus on the most influential annual study, conducted by NDARC. The Drug Trend Group at NDARC collects a significant set of data through its flag-ship project, the IDRS. Funded by the Australian Government's Department of Health and Ageing and the National Drug Law

Enforcement Research Fund since January 1997, the IDRS produces an annual report. The survey component of the IDRS sample is solely comprised of people who inject drugs.

Before canvassing some of the recent findings of the IDRS, it is first appropriate to unpack the language the report uses in the dissemination of results. The 2011 report explains that IRDS utilizes six distinct phrases to discuss pharmaceutical consumption among its sample: use of licitly obtained opioids; use of illicitly obtained opioids; use of any opioids; injection of licitly obtained opioids; injection of illicitly obtained opioids; and injection of any opioids (Stafford and Burns 2011). This language defines 'illicit' activity with pharmaceuticals in broad ways that are absent of contextual considerations. For instance, one report on IDRS data states that '"Licit" refers to drugs that were prescribed directly to the participant, while "illicit" refers to drugs that were directly prescribed to another person' (2012: 14). It is thus important to note that references to 'illicit acquisition' of pharmaceuticals include behaviors that may not typically constitute criminal activity. As well as indicating the purchase of pharmaceuticals 'on the street', the term 'illicit' may also encompass altered patterns of prescribed self-use and the use of pharmaceuticals prescribed to a friend or family member. Whether such an exchange with a friend or family member was voluntary is not considered. Use of the term 'illicit' here requires a significant assumption of deviance. As the IDRS literature moves seamlessly between references to acquisition and injection, observations about 'illicit use' of pharmaceuticals become blurred in the process.

As a data source for non-medical use, the IDRS disseminates the findings of survey questions about the price and availability of pharmaceuticals reported to be purchased 'illicitly'. The IDRS consistently reports that the most common method for the 'illicit acquisition' of methadone, buprenorphine, buprenorphine–naltrexone, morphine and oxycodone is through a friend—usually representing approximately half of the responses (Stafford and Breen 2016; Stafford and Burns 2011, 2012). The second most common method reported is through a 'known dealer', which amounts to approximately one quarter of the responses (Stafford and Breen 2016; Stafford and Burns 2011, 2012). According to the 2016, IDRS survey participants primarily reported that OST medications—methadone, buprenorphine and buprenorphine–naltrexone—were either 'easy' or 'very easy' to acquire 'illicitly' (Stafford and Breen 2016). Regarding prescription painkillers—morphine and oxycodone—only slightly less of the respondents reported 'easy' or 'very easy' access, while many more reported access as 'difficult' (Stafford and Breen 2016). Across all the pharmaceuticals investigated in the IDRS, a consistent observation has been the stability of an 'illicit supply' in street-based drug markets.

In the most recent survey, which comprised a sample of 888 people who inject drugs, 687 participants reported recent use an opiate, a number that has been consistently falling since 2012 (Stafford and Breen 2017). Morphine is the pharmaceutical most injected by the national sample (27%), as well as the pharmaceutical most commonly reported as the drug most injected in the month previous to data collection (Stafford and Breen 2017). When compared to heroin, morphine is, however, reported to be the drug 'most injected' substantially less; with 40% of the sample identifying heroin as the drug they injected most in the last month, while only 12% reported the same for morphine (Stafford and Breen 2017). It is also worth noting that 7% of the sample reported experiencing overdose related to an opiate other than heroin, while 42% reported experiencing an overdose related to heroin (Stafford and Breen 2017).

Due to a series of associated health concerns, there is a great deal of significance given to this kind of cataloging of reported rates. However, by focusing exclusively on injecting drug use there is a broad range of people who use opiates that are excluded from the IDRS sample. There is a standard line included in each IRDS report that acknowledges this: '*It is important to note that the results from the IDRS survey are not representative of injecting drug use in the general population*' (Stafford and Breen 2017: 1). Yet the association between injecting drug use and 'illicit consumption' is a powerful one in Australian culture, and its deeply moralized image often overshadows other forms of drug use (Moore 2004). In the case of non-medical use, the IDRS largely overlooks those who crush and snort their pharmaceuticals, or people who bite down on the drug, even those who let it dissolve under their tongue or just swallow it whole. This means that diverse forms of opiate consumption and the consumption of opiates among a diverse range of social and socioeconomic demographics are not being captured by IDRS data.

Police Detainees and DUMA

The second project that produces annual data about non-medical use is the Australian Institute of Criminology's (AIC) DUMA. In partnership with the AIC, state police services, and local researchers, a pilot version of DUMA was run in 1999, based on a similar system in the US. DUMA currently collects survey data and urine samples from police detainees (persons in police custody but not charged or convicted of a crime) on a quarterly basis, at nine sites across the country. Despite specific survey questions that impose a framework of 'abuse', a series of reports from the AIC have presented non-medical use as a problem that emerges 'naturally' from the data, as well as one that potentially impacts criminality.

Interpretations of DUMA data have produced observations about the majority of participants reporting that pharmaceuticals are either 'easy' or 'very easy' to obtain 'on the street' (Ng and Macgregor 2012). This is consistent with IDRS data, suggesting that pharmaceuticals are readily available in illicit drug markets. Yet little is known about how and from what sources medications are being diverted into illicit markets. Forged prescriptions and theft from medical facilities have been identified as contributing factors, but by no means account for how 'easy' detainees report their 'illicit acquisition' to be (Rodwell et al. 2010). It is, however, important to note that the most common response by survey participants was still that they acquire their pharmaceuticals from friends or acquaintances (Ng and Macgregor 2012).

The AIC also consistently report that non-medical use is more common among the DUMA sample than in the IDRS and broader population study samples, with female detainees commonly report higher rates of non-medical use than male detainees (McGregor et al. 2011). Benzodiazepine use in particular is thought to be highest among female detainees (Loxley 2007). This is largely consistent with data about women in prison reportedly having higher rates of drug use than their male counterparts (Butler et al. 2003; McClellan et al. 1997). It is, however, important to contextualize these findings by noting that samples of police detainees are not representative of either the general population or the criminal offending population.

Research suggests that the high visibility of disadvantaged populations in the criminal justice system means that they are more likely to come in contact with police and to spend more time in police custody (Smith and Visher 1981). Of particular controversy in Australia is the unequal time that Indigenous people spend detained in police custody uncharged (Cunneen 2005). Heavy alcohol use (Weatherburn 2008) and other forms of illicit (in particular injecting) drug use (Maher and Dixon 1999, 2001) also increase the likelihood and frequency of being detained by police. Moreover, the results of a survey conducted in the highly pressured environment of arrest must be approached with a degree of skepticism. The arrest and processing of detainees has also been described as an important element of the punishment of those accused of a crime (Feeley 1992). The potential for detainees to feel compelled to appear cooperative, and to produce answers that perform that cooperation is worth noting.

Given that social disadvantage shapes people's contact with the police, and the atmosphere of bewildered duress that characterizes the arrest process, it would seem rather unsurprising that AIC researchers found that:

> Among the detainees surveyed, more prescription drug users were unemployed, derived their income from welfare or benefits, considered themselves drug dependent, were currently on a drug-related charge and had been arrested or imprisoned in the previous 12 months by comparison with nonusers. (McGregor et al. 2011: 5)

Research suggests that samples of police detainees will be skewed toward very particular profiles of social disadvantage: thus it is clear that DUMA is not a generally representative sample of the Australian population. The project claims to provide information about connections between the criminal offending population and drug use, yet the data produced still only represent those who are in police custody, not people who have been convicted of a crime. While a collapsing of the categories of police detainee and convicted criminal is not explicit, the dissemination of DUMA data is suggestive of a link between non-medical use and criminal conduct.

As part of the project, DUMA also performs urinalysis tests on detainees who have apparently volunteered to participate. In the case of opiates, a positive urinalysis reading is sent for further testing to distinguish between heroin and other opiates (codeine and morphine). In a section analyzing urinalysis results and charges laid among detainees in the suburb of Bankstown, the authors of the 2009–2010 report write: 'Property offenders, drug offenders, road and traffic offenders and breach offenders all had higher rates of opiate use than benzodiazepine use. The opposite was true for violent [and] drink driving [offenders]' (Sweeney and Payne 2012: 46). The report presents a 'statistically significant' connection between positive urinalysis tests for opiates/benzodiazepines and criminal offences such as property damage, unsafe driving, violence and other forms of drug use. Claims about the connection between non-medical use and crime are, however, particularly limited because, as the methodological explanation of urinalysis in the report suggests, 'a positive result does not necessarily imply illicit use' (Sweeney and Payne 2012: 136).

References to 'illicit opiate use' are also particularly vague in much of the reporting of DUMA data. In a broader paper on drug use and property offending, Bradford and Payne name "self-reported days of illicit opioid use" (2012: 3) as a primary variable of interest. The paper defines 'illicit opioid use' as including "heroin, morphine, oxycodone, street methadone, or other illicit opioids" (Bradford and Payne 2012: 3). With definitions of 'illicit use' such as the ones described above, this literature suggests a conflation of what has previously been considered distinct medical and criminal forms of drug use. Decontextualized observations about non-medical use and 'illicit activity' are thus deployed in problematic ways in the DUMA literature. Though the collapsing of criminal and drug using behavior is by no means a new phenomenon, the vagueness with which projects such as DUMA refer to 'illicit pharmaceutical use' introduces a new area of concern about the potential to criminalize informal medication sharing and patient self-care.

National Data and the NDSHS

The necessity of large national projects that focus on 'illicit contexts' is consistently justified by the suggestion that they provide knowledge on a group that is of particular significance to the wider public. According to the NDARC website, the IDRS is "intended to serve as a strategic early warning system, identifying emerging trends of local and national concern in illicit drug markets" (Stafford and Breen 2016). Explanations of the project from a range of other institutions also tend to emphasis the 'strategic' nature of the project (Darke et al. 2000). One AIC report indicates that DUMA seeks to provide knowledge on the very specific cross section of 'drug users' and 'criminal offenders', because it is assumed that they 'have a greater impact on the quality of life of ordinary Australians than other groups of drug users' (Makkai 1999: 23). The language that surrounds explanations of both the IDRS and DUMA reveals a problematic emphasis on criminality, which is justified by presenting it as a 'strategic' focus on a population with 'greater impact' to the wider community.

Despite explanations of strategic value, the literature produced from the IDRS and DUMA seems to suggest a conflation of drug use and criminality. Though people who inject drugs and people who are alleged to have engaged in criminal activity are reasonable research foci, the "great majority of people who use drugs never come to the attention of doctors, lawyers, or policemen" (Robson 2009: 18). It is thus problematic that annual national data are only limited to criminalized contexts that are not representative of the wider drug using population.

The limitations of annual national data are not exclusive to the IDRS and DUMA. The National Drugs Strategy Household Survey (NDSHS) produces a tri-annual report funded by the Australian Institute of Health and Welfare that also provides a significant set of data on non-medical use. The NDSHS survey is sent out to a representative sample of more than 25,000 Australian households and comprises people aged 12 and older.

The most recent NDSHS reports have described a series of findings about the use of pharmaceuticals for non-medical purposes that have remained largely consistent. Of all the pharmaceuticals used for non-medical purposes, painkillers/analgesics are consistently found to be the drugs most likely for respondents to have consumed, followed by tranquillizers, barbiturates, benzodiazepines and sleeping pills (Australian Institute of Health and Welfare 2011, 2014, 2016). NDSHS data suggest that those who use painkillers/analgesics for non-medical purposes are most likely to be aged between 18 and 24 (Australian Institute of Health and Welfare 2016). There have also been slight variations in recent and lifetime use between genders in NDSHS data—men report higher rates of non-medical use over their lifetime, while recent use is reported as essentially the same across genders (Australian Institute of Health and Welfare 2008, 2011, 2014). According to the most recent NDSHS report (2016), 4.8% of the national sample used a pharmaceutical drug non-medially in the past 12 months, while 12.8% reported having ever used a pharmaceutical non-medically in their life.

Though the NDSHS does not provide as regular a set of data as the IDRS or DUMA, it does have a more general focus on the consumption of any drug, including alcohol. The NDSHS thus obviates some of the methodological limitations of national data collection. However, while a household sample does engage a broader cross section of people who use drugs, there are still limitations to worth noting.

The collection of NDSHS data is conducted under the banner of a study about 'drug use', a term that is largely associated with recreational or inebriate consumption. The perceived value of research into drug use seems tied to the assumption that such use is both a moral and health hazard. The 'illicit' perception of drug consumption is necessitated by a dominant moral code that constructs research into the practice to be proscriptive. Yet in many ways, pharmaceutical consumption is still thought of as 'safe', firmly embedded in medical conceptualizations of health. This provides a legitimizing framework that excludes even the term 'drug use' from the vocabulary of how most people think about the use of pharmaceuticals. Consequently, there is every likelihood that study respondents may not think of their consumption of painkillers as 'illicit' or part of the phenomena of 'drug use' that is the subject of the study.

National projects with such a significant quantitative focus are therefore unable to unpack and address the complexities of different types of consumption that blur the line between medical and non-medical, medicinal and recreational. Current national projects can only produce trend information about well-established populations of, what are often stigmatized communities of people who use drugs.

Diversion of Treatment Medications

Beyond national samples and surveillance studies, there has been a set of smaller-scale studies into non-medical use in Australia which have focused on the diversion, and the injection of OST medications (Larance et al. 2011; Winstock and Lea 2010; Winstock et al. 2007). OST drugs are prescribed to medically maintain the physiological components of opiate dependence—mainly withdrawal. Given that OST patients are necessarily already struggling with dependence-related issues, the non-medical use and diversion of their medication are likely to be higher than in other populations.

While research continues to suggest that the most common source of acquiring diverted OST medications is through friends and acquaintances (Larance et al. 2011), Australian studies suggest that, among those in buprenorphine treatment programs, approximately one-third claimed to have non-medically used their prescribed dose and/or have been involved in the diversion of their medication (Winstock et al. 2007). For buprenorphine–naloxone, it is closer to just over one-fifth of study respondents (Larance et al. 2011). Conversely, among those in a methadone program (the most popular OST available in Australia) only a little over one-tenth say that they have used the drug non-medically or have been involved in its diversion (Winstock and Lea 2010).

Research into the injection and/or diversion of OST medications is focused on the harms and potential harms that surround the practice. Buprenorphine in particular has been identified as the OST drug most likely to be diverted (Winstock et al. 2007). Still, the harms associated with the injection of OST medications remain tied to a sample of people already embedded in criminal networks. In a 2005 study into the diversion of buprenorphine in Melbourne, the authors conclude that 'recent buprenorphine injection was associated with the injection of other drug types, injection-related health problems, opioid substitution treatment and involvement in crime' (Jenkinson et al. 2005: 200).

Criminal activity is often included as one of the health concerns identified in this body of research, with little critical discussion of how structural and policy frameworks that criminalize people who inject drugs. A recent body of research has emphasized the importance of environmental factors associated with the harms of injecting drug use and includes those produced by its criminalization (Strathdee et al. 2010; Rhodes 2002). However, literature about environmental interventions has paid less attention to the way criminalized cultures of injecting drug use affect the intravenous use of pharmaceuticals.

While an emphasis on intravenous use of treatment medications is entirely appropriate when studying patients in OST, there is a range of methods of painkiller administration for which data are scarce. Australian research focuses on samples of people who inject drugs or on criminalized contexts in which injecting drug use is more common. The data's broad focus on injecting use is unlikely to be representative of non-medical painkiller consumption in Australia. A lack of representative data about the range of practices that comprise non-medical use in Australia may be presenting a disproportionate image of pathology and criminality to those required to respond to non-medical consumption as a public health concern.

Policy Responses to Non-Medical Use

In January 2006, the Drugs and Crime Prevention Committee of the Victorian Parliament was asked to conduct an inquiry into the nature, extent and culture of the non-medical use of benzodiazepines and other pharmaceuticals in Victoria. In the final report, which was delivered in March 2007, the 'Forward', written by the chair of the committee Judy Maddigan, states:

> The most telling part of our investigations was the realisation that many people within the community do not perceive prescription drug abuse to be a form of drug abuse. Consequently, they are unaware of the harms that are associated with the misuse and abuse of prescription medications... Challenging the culture of drug use and abuse and contesting ideas as to what does or does not count as a 'drug' is a very difficult task. (Drugs and Crime Prevention Committee 2007: 2)

This model of concern about a hidden but growing problem of medication 'abuse' set the stage for many of the policy responses to come. The regulation of pharmaceuticals being used non-medically was given national coverage after the Victorian Coroner John Olle subsequently called for a public health response in the form of real-time monitoring of pharmaceutical purchases. In early 2012, Olle remarked:

> Where prescription shoppers are identified, they should in the first instance be directed to support services, with law enforcement only involved with persistent shoppers and/or those who are motivated by profit rather than drug dependence. (Dearne 2012a)

Olle's remarks sparked debate about the appropriate policy response. This section discusses a range of trial and proposed monitoring systems to address the diversion and non-medical consumption of pharmaceuticals, as well as some initial regulatory changes. It starts by addressing a 2005 pharmacy level amphetamine monitoring system called Project STOP which served as a forerunner to a broader Tasmanian system that has been recommended for a national roll-out, and finally outlines recent changes to availability of codeine-containing products.

One of the first campaigns to address issues surrounding non-medical use in Australia was the Pharmacy Guild of Australia's 'Project STOP'. Project STOP began on a trial basis in Queensland in November of 2005, before rolling-out a national scheme soon after. The initiative provided participating pharmacies with real-time monitoring of an individual's purchases of products containing pseudoephedrine. Project STOP places a focus on the use of certain pharmaceuticals as precursors for the manufacture of illicit drugs, maintaining conceptual distance between licit and illicit forms of the drug. The project claims to provide pharmacists with a tool to negotiate the therapeutic needs of their clients, and in turn to determine whether they will sell to the customer (Pharmacy Guild of Australia 2007). It is significant to note that Project STOP emerged in a heighten political atmosphere which was responding to hyperbolic media coverage about methamphetamine use as a 'new drug epidemic' (Ritter 2007). As part of apparent efforts to address the 'amphetamine problem', a set of supply-side, prohibitionist oriented policy initiatives were introduced in the mid-2000s (Groves and Marmo 2009), of which Project STOP was part.

In 2012, the first real-time monitoring system for all pharmaceutical purchases was rolled out across Tasmania. Developed as part of the state's Drugs and Poisons Information System, pharmacists were required to register clients and their purchases through Online Remote Access (DORA) software. Though DORA was applied to a broader range of pharmaceuticals, it was largely based on the software used for Project STOP. It is worth noting that the shadow of a moral panic about a 'new epidemic' of 'illicit drug abuse' informed the first response to issues surrounding the diversion of pharmaceuticals, and the foundation of a proposed national system.

Unlike Project STOP, however, Tasmania's DORA system was presented as a tool to identify 'doctor shopping' and 'diversion', as well as to address the potential for non-medical pharmaceutical use. The DORA system has even been presented as an initiative in Australia's apparent 'war on drugs'. In a radio segment for 936 ABC, Hobart titled 'Tasmania taking the lead in the war on drugs' the program was introduced as follows: "The latest illicit drug trade may be right under your nose and Tasmania is taking the lead in tackling it" (Brown 2012). In early 2013, then Federal Health Minister Tanya Plibersek announced 5 million dollars of funding for the establishment of a national system for the Electronic Recording and Reporting of Controlled Drugs (ERRCD) that was to be based on the DORA system (Dearne 2012b). In response to three overdose deaths in a period of three months in rural NSW, the Australian Medical Association reiterated the apparent urgency of a national roll-out (Kaye 2013).

There is, however, several potentially problematic elements of this kind of register and track approach that state and federal governments seem invested in. The registration of pharmacy clients and their purchases has the potential to act as a punitive form of social control. An assumed advantage of the system is that clients wanting to avoid registered purchases will be encouraged to pursue alternative treatments for pain relief. Yet this touted benefit ignores the related implication that clients may opt for lower potency pharmaceuticals and therefore have less effective therapeutic outcomes, in an attempt to avoid registered purchases. Patients may also feel encouraged to alter the prescribed use of medications that are more difficult to acquire.

An important comparison is also found in the way registered clients and monitored purchases might resemble aspects of the concept of 'liquid handcuffs', which is used to describe the overly punitive elements of some methadone services (Smith 2011). Several methadone services attach a range of conditions to access to the medication that impose models of discipline on the client. Some methadone prescribers do not allow clients to collect their dose accompanied by friends or family members and reserve the right to refuse sale if the client is not presented appropriately (i.e., neat clothing and grooming) (Fraser and Valentine 2008). The potential for similar restrictions on other medications monitored under the proposed system is worth noting. Lastly, unnecessary monitoring may potentially result in those simply altering their medical treatment being funneled into drug treatment programs. Misunderstandings between clients and dispensers about the nature of multiple prescriptions may identify a range of 'serial shoppers' that, under the proposed ERRCD, prescribers and dispensers' will have little choice but to refer to law enforcement.

If a national roll-out of the ERRCD proceeds, this will formalize the discourses of 'abuse' and 'illicit' activity that dominate the literature about non-medical consumption. The potential to transform creative medication consumption into a 'substance use problem' requiring treatment, as well as the possibility of criminalizing consumers who resist problems in the system, is important to consider. Much like the research literature canvassed throughout the chapter, the kinds of responses outlined in this section reveal a trajectory of prohibitionist policies that are likely to pathologize and criminalize the people who come in contact with them.

Despite much lobbying for real-time monitoring by representative bodies of pharmacies, this approach has now been largely rejected by the Therapeutic Goods Administration (TGA). The TGA has instead opted to address the availability of codeine-containing medication over-the-counter by rescheduling these drugs from schedules 2 or 3, making them all schedule 4 medications: meaning that a prescription is now required to acquire them. In response to criticism from key pharmaceutical groups such as the Australian Self Medication Industry, the TGA's chief medical officer Tim Greenway has been recently reported in the media as saying 'It's important that people realise that the decision's been taken based on safety predominantly and based on the risk of abuse' (Conifer and Keany 2016). While changes to the scheduling of codeine may change the landscape of over-the-counter consumption, the way policymakers will address concerns about the potential harms of prescription pain medications remains to be seen.

Conclusion

This chapter has outlined the emergence of a discourse of 'abuse' surrounding non-medical consumption. It has explored how a range of research communities have sought to make scientific claim on the practice of non-medical consumption, purporting to have 'discovered' and begun to 'measure' a 'new drug problem'. The construction of this 'new drug problem' is informed by data that often conflates practices of informal medication sharing with the intention to divert medications into illicit markets. While research communities have demonstrated an apparent consensus on use of a discourse of abuse to describe non-medical consumption, there is less consensus on the meaning and measurement of this 'abuse'.

Thus far the book has demonstrated the social and political formation of discourses about drugs and their 'misuse' or 'abuse'. The previous chapter outlined the social history of Australia's approach to drugs and the unstable distinctions it formed between 'licit' and 'illicit' forms of opiates. This chapter outlined a shift in the way this distinction is produced, revealing a preoccupation with medical authority, psychological dysfunction and criminality. Through attempts to reproduce the importance of medical compliance, 'illicit' and pathologized enactments of the painkiller now form the foundation of research literature about non-medical consumption. However, this literature has ignored the social significance of the specific drugs being consumed and the context in which they are used.

Part II of the book will address these gaps in the literature through an empirical investigation into a range of contexts of painkiller consumption. Before arriving at an empirical assessment of user perspectives, it is, however, useful to engage in one more exercise of historical and discursive analysis. The next chapter will explore cultural understandings of pain and the social meanings attached to the consumption of pain medications.

References

American Psychiatric Association. (2013). *Diagnostic and Statistical Manual of Mental Disorders: DSM-5*. Arlington: American Psychiatric Publication.

Arria, A. M., Garnier-Dykstra, L. M., Caldeira, K. M., Vincent, K. B., & O'Grady, K. E. (2011). Prescription Analgesic Use Among Young Adults: Adherence to Physician Instructions and Diversion. *Pain Medicine, 12*(6), 898–903.

Australian Institute of Health and Welfare. (2008). *National Drugs Strategy Household Survey: Detailed Findings* (Drug Statistics Series No. 22). Australian Government.

Australian Institute of Health and Welfare. (2011). *National Drugs Strategy Household Survey: Detailed Findings* (Drug Statistics Series No. 25). Australian Government.

Australian Institute of Health and Welfare. (2014). *National Drugs Strategy Household Survey: Detailed Findings* (Drug Statistics Series No. 28). Australian Government.

Australian Institute of Health and Welfare. (2016). *National Drugs Strategy Household Survey: Detailed Findings* (Drug Statistics Series No. 31). Australian Government.

Becker, W. C., Sullivan, L. E., Tetrault, J. M., Desai, R. A., & Fiellin, D. A. (2008). Non-Medical Use, Abuse and Dependence on Prescription Opioids Among U.S. Adults: Psychiatric, Medical and Substance Use Correlates. *Drug and Alcohol Dependence, 94*(1–3), 38–47.

Bradford, D., & Payne, J. (2012). Illicit Drug Use and Property Offending Among Police Detainees. *Contemporary Issues in Crime and Justice, 157,* 1–12.

Brown, D. (2012). *Tasmania Taking the Lead in the War on Drugs*. Retrieved August 17, 2011, from http://blogs.abc.net.au/tasmania/2012/06/tasmania-taking-the-lead-in-the-war-on-drug.

Butler, T., Levy, M., Dolan, K., & Kaldor, J. (2003). Drug Use and Its Correlates in an Australian Prisoner Population. *Addiction Research & Theory, 11*(2), 89–101.

Catalano, J. (2009). Pain Management and Substance Abuse: A National Dilemma. *Social Work in Public Health, 24*(6), 477–490.

Compton, W. M., & Volkow, N. D. (2006a). Abuse of Prescription Drugs and the Risk of Addiction. *Drug and Alcohol Dependence, 83,* S4–S7.

Compton, W. M., & Volkow, N. D. (2006b). Major Increases in Opioid Analgesic Abuse in the United States: Concerns and Strategies. *Drug and Alcohol Dependence, 81*(2), 103–107.

Conifer, D., & Keany, F. (2016, December 20). Painkillers with Codeine Won't Be Available Over the Counter from 2018. *ABC News*.

Cunneen, C. (2005). Racism, Discrimination and the Over-Representation of Indigenous People in the Criminal Justice System: Some Conceptual and Explanatory Issues. *Current Issues in Criminal Justice, 17*(3), 329–346.

Darke, S., Hall, W., & Topp, L. (2000). *The Illicit Drug Reporting System (IDRS) 1996–2000: History and Development of a National Strategic Early Warning System for Monitoring Trends in Illicit Drug Use*. Sydney: National Drug and Alcohol Research Centre, UNSW.

Davey, P. J., Ramm, R. A., Ball, A. R., & Wilks, J. (1995). A Profile of Therapeutic Opioid Dependent Persons in Queensland. *Australian Health Review, 18*(3), 76–90.

Dearne, K. (2012a, April 14). Electronic Alert to End Abuse. *The Australian*.

Dearne, K. (2012b, April 21). Plibersek Defends Script Alert System. *The Australian*.

Degenhardt, L., Larance, B., Mathers, B., Azim, T., Kamarulzaman, A., Mattick, R., et al. (2007). *Benefits and Risks of Pharmaceutical Opioids: Essential Treatment and Diverted Medication. A Global Review of Availability,*

Extra-Medical Use, Injection and the Association with HIV. Reference Group to the United Nations on HIV and Injecting Drug Use. Sydney: National Drug and Alcohol Research Centre, UNSW.

Drugs and Crime Prevention Committee. (2007). *Inquiry into the Misuse/Abuse of Benzodiazepines and Other Forms of Pharmaceutical Drugs in Victoria* (Final Report). Parliament of Victoria.

Dyson, T. (1992). Sexual Behaviour and Networking: Anthropological and Socio-Cultural Studies on the Transmission of HIV. *Journal of Epidemiology Community Health, 48*(2), 214.

Feeley, M. (1992). *The Process Is the Punishment: Handling Cases in a Lower Criminal Court*. New York: Russell Sage Foundation.

Fischer, M. A., Stedman, M. R., Lii, J., Vogeli, C., Shrank, W. H., Brookhart, M. A., et al. (2010). Primary Medication Non-Adherence: Analysis of 195,930 Electronic Prescriptions. *Journal of General Internal Medicine, 25*(4), 284–290.

Fraser, S., & Valentine, K. (2008). *Substance and Substitution: Methadone Subjects in Liberal Societies*. Basingstoke: Palgrave Macmillan.

Fraser, S., Moore, D., & Keane, H. (2014). *Habits: Remaking Addiction*. Basingstoke: Palgrave Macmillan.

Groves, A., & Marmo, M. (2009). How to 'Melt the Ice' on the Streets: A Social-Control Analysis on the Rise of Methamphetamine Within Australia and the Need to Reduce Demand. *Current Issues in Criminal Justice, 20*(3), 413–432.

Inciardi, J. A., Surratt, H. L., Cicero, T. J., & Beard, R. A. (2009). Prescription Opioid Abuse and Diversion in an Urban Community: The Results of an Ultrarapid Assessment. *Pain Medicine, 10*(3), 537–548.

Jenkinson, R. A., Clark, N. C., Fry, C. L., & Dobbin, M. (2005). Buprenorphine Diversion and Injection in Melbourne, Australia: An Emerging Issue? *Addiction, 100*(2), 197–205.

Kaye, B. (2013). *AMA Repeats Calls for DORA National Roll-Out*. Retrieved July 30, 2013, from http://www.medicalobserver.com.au/news/ama-repeats-calls-for-dora-national-rollout.

Keane, H. (2011). Drugs That Work: Pharmaceuticals and Performance Self-Management. In S. Fraser & D. Moore (Eds.), *The Drug Effect: Health, Crime and Society*. Cambridge: Cambridge University Press.

Keane, H., Moore, D., & Fraser, S. (2011). Addiction and Dependence: Making Realities in the DSM. *Addiction, 106*(5), 875–877.

Kelly, B. C., & Parsons, J. T. (2007). Prescription Drug Misuse Among Club Drug-Using Young Adults. *American Journal of Drug and Alcohol Abuse, 33*(6), 875–884.

Kirsh, K. L., Jass, C., Bennett, D. S., Hagen, J. E., & Passik, S. D. (2007). Initial Development of a Survey Tool to Detect Issues of Chemical Coping in Chronic Pain Patients. *Palliative and Supportive Care, 5*(3), 219–226.

Kwon, J. H., Tanco, K., Hui, D., Reddy, A., & Bruera, E. (2014). Chemical Coping Versus Pseudoaddiction in Patients with Cancer Pain. *Palliative and Supportive Care, 12*(5), 1–5.

Larance, B., Degenhardt, L., Lintzeris, N., Winstock, A., & Mattick, R. (2011). Definitions Related to the Use of Pharmaceutical Opioids: Extramedical Use, Diversion, Non-Adherence and Aberrant Medication-Related Behaviours. *Drug and Alcohol Review, 30*(3), 236–245.

Littlejohn, C., Baldacchino, A., & Bannister, J. (2004). Chronic Non-Cancer Pain and Opioid Dependence. *Journal of the Royal Society of Medicine, 97*(2), 62–65.

Loxley, W. (2007). *Benzodiazepine Use and Harms Among Police Detainees in Australia* (Trends & Issues in Crime and Criminal Justice No. 336). Canberra: Australian Institute of Criminology.

Maher, L., & Dixon, D. (1999). Policing and Public Health: Law Enforcement and Harm Minimization in a Street-Level Drug Market. *British Journal of Criminology, 39*(4), 488–512.

Maher, L., & Dixon, D. (2001). Cost of Crackdowns: Policing Cabramatta'S Heroin Market. *Current Issues in Criminal Justice, 13*(1), 5–22.

Makkai, T. (1999). *Drug Use Monitoring in Australia. A Brief Description* (Research and Public Policy Series No. 21). Canberra: Australian Institute of Criminology.

McClellan, D. S., Farabee, D., & Crouch, B. M. (1997). Early Victimization, Drug Use, and Criminality: A Comparison of Male and Female Prisoners. *Criminal Justice and Behavior, 24*(4), 455–476.

McGregor, C., Gately, N., & Fleming, J. (2011). *Prescription Drug Use Among Detainees: Prevalence, Sources and Links to Crime* (Trends & Issues in Crime and Criminal Justice No. 423). The Australian Institute of Criminology.

Moore, D. (2004). Governing Street-Based Injecting Drug Users: A Critique of Heroin Overdose Prevention in Australia. *Social Science and Medicine, 59*(7), 1547–1557.

Moore, D. (2008). Erasing Pleasure from Public Discourse on Illicit Drugs: On the Creation and Reproduction of an Absence. *International Journal of Drug Policy, 19*(5), 353–358.

National Drug and Alcohol Research Centre. (2012). Key Findings: Drug Trend Conference Handout Australian. *Drug Trends 2012, Findings from the Illicit Drug Reporting System.*

Ng, S., & Macgregor, S. (2012). *Pharmaceutical Drug Use Among Police Detainees* (Research in Practice No. 23). Canberra: Australian Institute of Criminology.

Passik, S. D., & Kirsh, K. L. (2004). Assessing Aberrant Drug-Taking Behaviors in the Patient with Chronic Pain. *Current Pain and Headache Reports, 8*(4), 289–294.

Pharmacy Guild of Australia. (2007). *Project STOP*. Retrieved August 17, 2011, from www.projectstop.com.au/.

Pradel, V., Delga, C., Rouby, F., Micallef, J., & Lapeyre-Mestre, M. (2010). Assessment of Abuse Potential of Benzodiazepines from a Prescription Database Using 'Doctor Shopping' as an Indicator. *CNS Drugs, 24*(7), 611–620.

Rhodes, T. (2002). The 'Risk Environment': A Framework for Understanding and Reducing Drug-Related Harm. *International Journal of Drug Policy, 13*(2), 85–94.

Rhodes, T., Singer, M., Bourgois, P., Friedman, S. R., & Strathdee, S. A. (2005). The Social Structural Production of HIV Risk Among Injecting Drug Users. *Social Science and Medicine, 61*(5), 1026–1044.

Ritter, A. (2007). Methamphetamine Alarm: Are We Forgetting What We Know? *Drug and Alcohol Review, 26*(3), 227–230.

Ritter, A., & Natale, R. D. (2005). The Relationship Between Take-Away Methadone Policies and Methadone Diversion. *Drug and Alcohol Review, 24*(4), 347–352.

Robson, P. (2009). *Forbidden Drugs*. Oxford: Oxford University Press.

Rodwell, L., Ringland, C., & Bradford, D. (2010). What Do Police Data Tell Us About Criminal Methods of Obtaining Prescription Drugs? *Contemporary Issues in Crime and Justice, 139,* 1–12.

Sees, K., Di Marino, M. E., Ruediger, N. K., Sweeney, C. T., & Shiffman, S. (2005). Non-Medical Use of OxyContin Tablets in the United States. *Journal of Pain & Palliative Care Pharmacotherapy., 19*(2), 13–23.

Smith, C. B. (2011). A Users' Guide to 'Juice Bars' and 'Liquid Handcuffs' Fluid Negotiations of Subjectivity, Space and the Substance of Methadone Treatment. *Space and Culture, 14*(3), 291–309.

Smith, D. A., & Visher, C. A. (1981). Street-Level Justice: Situational Determinants of Police Arrest Decisions. *Social Problems, 29*(2), 167–177.

Stafford, J., & Breen, C. (2016). *Australian Drug Trends 2015: Findings from the Illicit Drug Reporting System (IDRS)* (Australian Drug Trend Series No. 145). Sydney: National Drug and Alcohol Research Centre, UNSW.

Stafford, J., & Breen, C. (2017). *Australian Drug Trends 2017: Preliminary Findings from the Illicit Drug Reporting System (IDRS)*. Sydney: National Drug and Alcohol Research Centre, UNSW.

Stafford, J., & Burns, L. (2011). *Australian Drug Trends 2010: Findings from the Illicit Drug Reporting System (IDRS)* (Australian Drug Trends Series No. 73). Sydney: National Drug and Alcohol Research Centre, UNSW.

Stafford, J., & Burns, L. (2012). *Australian Drug Trends 2011: Findings from the Illicit Drug Reporting System (IDRS)* (Australian Drug Trends Series No. 91). Sydney: National Drug and Alcohol Research Centre, UNSW.

Strathdee, S. A., Hallett, T. B., Bobrova, N., Rhodes, T., Booth, R., Abdool, R., et al. (2010). HIV and Risk Environment for Injecting Drug Users: The Past, Present, and Future. *Lancet, 376*(9737), 268–284.

Sweeney, J., & Payne, J. (2012). *Drug Use Monitoring in Australia: 2009–10 Report on Drug Use Among Police Detainees AIC Reports* (Monitoring Reports 17). Australian Institute of Criminology.

Treloar, C., & Holt, M. (2006). Deficit Models and Divergent Philosophies: Service Providers' Perspectives on Barriers and Incentives to Drug Treatment. *Drugs: Education, Prevention, and Policy, 13*(4), 367–382.

Vivian, J., Saleheen, H., Singer, M., Navarro, J., & Mirhej, G. (2005). Under the Counter: The Diffusion of Narcotic Analgesics to the Inner City Street. *Journal of Ethnicity in Substance Abuse, 4*(2), 97–114.

Volkow, N. D., Fowler, J. S., Wang, G.-J., & Swanson, J. M. (2004). Dopamine in Drug Abuse and Addiction: Results from Imaging Studies and Treatment Implications. *Molecular Psychiatry, 9*(6), 557–569.

Weatherburn, D. J. (2008). The Role of Drug and Alcohol Policy in Reducing Indigenous Over-Representation in Prison. *Drug and Alcohol Review, 27*(1), 91–94.

Webster, L. R., & Webster, R. M. (2005). Predicting Aberrant Behaviors in Opioid-Treated Patients: Preliminary Validation of the Opioid Risk Tool. *Pain Medicine, 6*(6), 432–442.

Winstock, A. R., & Lea, T. (2010). Diversion and Injection of Methadone and Buprenorphine Among Clients in Public Opioid Treatment Clinics in New South Wales, Australia. *Substance Use & Misuse, 45*(1–2), 240–252.

Winstock, A. R., Lea, T., & Sheridan, J. (2007). Prevalence of Diversion and Injection of Methadone and Buprenorphine Among Clients Receiving Opioid Treatment at Community Pharmacies in New South Wales, Australia. *International Journal of Drug Policy, 19*(6), 450–458.

World Health Organization. (2013). *International Classification of Diseases (ICD)*. Retrieved June 4, 2011, from http://www.who.int/classifications/icd/en/.

4

Problematizing Pain: Medical, Social and Commercial Approaches to Pain

Pain is a universal human experience. It is an inalienable part of the human condition. The sensation that accompanies bruised or torn flesh is instantly recognizable. The stress of a busy day and the painful throb of a headache are a common part of contemporary life. The way people relieve pain is almost as recognizable. It usually comes in the form of a pill, bought over-the-counter or prescribed by the doctor. Nurofen® and Panadol® are household brands that can be found in most handbags and briefcases, kitchen cabinets and staff cupboards alike. Those who have been admitted to hospital, or have visited a friend or family member there, will be familiar with the catheter drip of morphine. Once discharged, the takeaway prescription is usually OxyContin® or Endone®. Like pain, painkillers are a mundane part of everyday life. Though it is a common human experience, pain is not often well understood. Medical definitions most often relate to physical injury, while colloquial uses of the term encompass a much broader set of experiences of human suffering. The way pain is defined, experienced and understood is thus influenced by the conditions under which it is felt as well as the discourses used to articulate it. This chapter considers pain from three key

G. C. Dertadian, *A Fine Line*,
https://doi.org/10.1007/978-981-13-1975-4_4

vantage points: as an issue within medical inquiry and treatment, as the main concern of an emerging field of specialist pain medicine and as an expanding and increasingly commercialized category of discomfort and suffering in late-modernity.

Thus far, Part I of this book has articulated the social construction of distinctions between kinds of opiates (and other drugs), and the political and professional interests that have informed them. Chapter 2 outlined the significance of international influences and the prominence of the medical profession in the historical development of 'licit' and 'illicit' forms of opiate. Produced under a discourse about the 'therapeutic' or 'abusive' potential of each drug, medical authority became an important element of their continued symbolic separation throughout the twentieth century. Chapter 3 described a shift in the way these distinctions, between the 'licit' and 'illicit' capacity of drugs, are being formulated in the twenty-first century. Among the contest of epidemiological, psychological and medical perspectives that have attempted to formulate a scientific body of research about non-medical consumption, the practice is largely regarded as 'abusive' and thus as representative of a psychological or criminal pathology.

Whereas the previous chapters have contextualized the social and political histories that have informed drug consumption and the knowledge produced around it, this chapter focuses specifically on pain, its treatment, stigmatization and commercialization. It asks how contemporary understandings of pain contribute to the social, political and discursive context in which painkillers are consumed. The chapter starts by exploring the way general medicine conceptualizes pain, before moving to discuss the emergence of the field of pain medicine and its approach to the neurology of the pain patient. It also explores the way neurological accounts from pain medicine have informed debates about 'addiction' and the social and emotional influences on chronic pain. The chapter also draws on theory from sociology and cultural studies to elaborate on the significance of the body and governance of the self as it relates to contemporary understandings of pain. This literature is used to consider the blurring boundaries between pain, anxiety and discomfort in consumer culture.

General Medicine and Analgesic Medications

The diagnosis and treatment of pain-related symptoms and disorders form one of the most contested areas of modern medicine. Among an array of contentious elements, the medical community seems to have come to the consensus that pain can be broadly divided into two categories: acute and chronic. Acute pain is most often defined by "its distinct onset, obvious cause, and short duration", while chronic pain is usually defined by "its persistence beyond an expected time frame for healing" (Ferrell 2003: 323–324). Chronic pain is a more complex phenomenon that is often regarded as difficult to treat. The specialty of pain medicine has shaped and been shaped by this distinction between acute and chronic pain. Rising interest in chronic pain within the medical profession, and the frameworks used to diagnose and treatment it, will be taken up in more detail in the next section. Aside from pain medicine's specific interest in chronic pain, general medicine is typically concerned with acute pain.

In general medicine, acute pain is understood as a "warning system, as our body's attempt to draw attention to a body part that has been injured or that is in danger" (Northern Private Pain Centre 2012). Most general medical practitioners who encounter acute pain thus understand it to be caused by another underlying medical issue. A focus on correcting the underlying medical issue is taken in the informed hope that the pain will disappear accordingly: broken bones cause pain that fades as the bone heals; high fevers cause pain that diminishes as the fever subsides. The most common medical response to acute pain is the recommendation or prescription of analgesic medications within a given timeframe. Within Australia, patent guidelines and Federal and State legislation regulate the availability of analgesic medications for prescription by physicians and over-the-counter purchase by consumers.

Established under the *Therapeutic Goods Act 1989*, the scheduling of drugs in Australia is overseen by the National Drugs and Poisons Schedule Committee (NDPSC). All Australian states and territories adopt the substantive component of the scheduling system set out by the NDPSC, though slight jurisdictional variations do exist (Royal

Australasian College of Physicians 2009). An assortment of low-dose paracetamol and ibuprofen codeine products used to be classified as Schedule 2 Pharmacy Medicines, while higher-dose formulations of these substances, like Panadeine Extra® (paracetamol and codeine phosphate) and Mersyndol® (paracetamol, codeine phosphate, doxylamine succinate), were considered Schedule 3 Pharmacist Only Medicines. All medication containing codeine have now been grouped with medication such as Tylenol® (co-codamol) and Tramadol® (hydrochloride capsules), which are classified as Schedule 4 Prescription Only Medications: requiring professional medical monitoring. However, most opiate (and analgesic) formulations are classified as Schedule 8 Controlled Substances, whose possession without permission is a criminal offence. Under NDPSC regulation 'permission' for access to Schedule 8 opiates can only be granted by a medical practitioner and for 'therapeutic purposes'.

One final opiate formulation called diacetylmorphine, commonly known as heroin, is a Schedule 9 Prohibited Substance. The sale, distribution, use and manufacture (except for the purposes of research) of Schedule 9 substances is prohibited by law. While diacetylmorphine is prohibited in Australia, it is available for analgesic purposes, such as the relief of chronic and malignant pain, in the UK and elsewhere (Van de Werf et al. 2003). Medical research about the analgesic capacity of diacetylmorphine is, however, limited, with much of the medical literature focusing on its uses as a replacement therapy for people who have been in treatment for chronic relapsing opiate dependence (Clark 2010; Nosyk et al. 2012).

Medical literature about analgesic medications primarily focuses on opiates. This literature divides opiates into three categories: opioid agonists, opioid antagonists and opioid agonist–antagonists. Examples of opioid agonists include oxycodone and methadone. Opioid agonists are described as substances that attach themselves to and activate opioid receptors in the brain, which is what is thought to produce the analgesic effect (Berger 2005). The activation of opioid receptors in the brain is the same neurological process that can result in the pleasurable or euphoric feeling of the opiate 'high' (Robson 2009). Though a distinction is often made between the therapeutic qualities of analgesia, and the pleasurable qualities of an opiate 'high', little explanation about what makes them distinct is provided in the medical literature. It is worth noting that this may be linked to a general avoidance of discussion of pleasure in drug research (Fraser 2008).

What explanations that do exist in the medical literature tend to describe the presence of physical pain and its alleviation through the activation of opioid receptors as what characterizes the process of analgesia. Explanations of the neurology of pain and its subsequent interaction with analgesic medication are not well developed in the literature. Rather than any neurological explanation about the assumed difference between analgesia and pleasurable inebriation, the literature relies on descriptions about physical suffering and its alleviation through the activation of opioid receptors.

On the other hand, explanations of opioid antagonists tend to describe a chemical substance that also attach to opioid receptors but do not activate these receptors. Opioid antagonists therefore block or reverse the effects of analgesia and respiratory depression. Opioid antagonists like naltrexone and naloxone are most often recommended for overdose prevention (Sporer and Kral 2007). The last opioid category, opioid agonist–antagonists, are thought to attach to the same opioid receptors, activating some, while blocking others. Drugs such as nalbuphine and buprenorphine are considered agonist–antagonists and descriptions of their use relate mostly to mild analgesia with limited respiratory depression and low levels of tolerance building (Stoelting and Hillier 2012).

The principles that guide general medical approaches to pain are tied closely to the medications used to treat it. Legislative regulation and scientific accounts of analgesic medications often refer to their appropriateness for the relief of acute and/or chronic pain. While pain relief is a common part of general practice, it is largely described as peripheral to the central role of general medicine, whose primary objective is to address the underlying condition. This is, however, not the case with chronic pain. Though the medical practitioner may often know the origins of chronic pain, the ongoing cause is rarely identifiable. The specialty of pain medicine came about largely as a result of rising interest in chronic pain and has developed tensions with medical approaches to pain more broadly.

The Evolution of Pain Medicine

The medical profession has long been concerned with an appropriate language to 'measure' pain (Meldrum 2003). In a 1939 study, Dallenbach developed a series of 44 terms that attempted to categorize the temporal, spatial, pleasurable, affective and qualitative attributes of pain. In 1971, researchers at McGill University in Montreal recruited a panel of students, patients and doctors to refine Dallenbach's classification of pain terms. The McGill Pain Scale, as it came to be known, divided the terms used to describe pain into three categories: sensory, affective and evaluative (Melzack 1975). The medical profession has since developed a range of other tools to 'measure' levels of pain including verbal, visual and numerical rating scales (Frampton and Hughes-Webb 2011).

Despite a proliferation of tools of measurement, little consensus has emerged on the reliability of any one system of pain measurement and the medical literature consistently comments upon the difficulty of its study and treatment:

> Progress in measurement has been slow because pain is a complex perceptual experience that can be quantified only indirectly. (Chapman et al. 1985: 1)

> ...attempts to make valid assessments of [pain] have been fraught with difficulties. (Briggs and Closs 1999: 438)

> Although certain physiological responses or behaviors prompted by pain may be observed, modern medicine has produced no single parameter to represent our understanding of what we know to be pain. (Noble et al. 2005: 14)

The medical profession broadly views pain scales as problematic because of the supposed unreliability of a patient's subjective self-evaluation, at least as in comparison with ostensibly externally verifiable methods of testing such as biopsy or necropsy.

The development of the field of pain medicine has, however, been less concerned with the capacity to accurately measure pain. Pain medicine developed rapidly as a field distinct from general medicine after a 1965 publication by Melzack and Wall that presented pain not only as the result of disease or trauma but as a medical problem in itself (1967). In this influential publication, Melzack and Wall describe how the transmission of messages about pain to the brain could be both obstructed and facilitated by mechanisms in the dorsal horns of the spine. The gate control theory, as it came to be known, demonstrated that the transmission of such messages was based on the 'active peripheral fibers, as well as the dynamic action of the brain process. As a result, psychological variables such as past experience, attention, and other cognitive activities have been integrated into current research and therapy on pain processes' (Melzack 1996: 128). The significance of the gate control theory was that it challenged medicine's then dualistic model of pain as either the body's proportional response to tissue damage or the individual's imagined experience (Meldrum 2003).

Following the gate control theory the field adopted the perspective that pain is an 'experience which can be reported only by the sufferer' (Noble et al. 2005: 14). In 1979, the International Association for the Study of Pain (IASP) developed the following definition, which is still in use today: "[pain is] an unpleasant sensory and emotional experience, associated with actual or potential tissue damage, or described in terms of such damage" (IASP 2014). Due in large part to the development of the specialty of pain medicine, the medical profession more broadly began to acknowledge that pain is not merely a naturally occurring object that can be measured.

In March 2010, more than two hundred representatives from various health, consumer and industry groups gathered for the first time in Australian (and international) history, for the explicit purpose of finding ways to improve the assessment and treatment of pain. The National Pain Summit, as it was referred to, produced a report that was to act as a guideline for the future of the specialty of pain medicine. The authors of the report reiterate the notion that pain is only subjectively verifiable:

'all pain is an individual human experience that is entirely subjective and that can only be truly appreciated by the individual experiencing the pain' (National Pain Summit Initiative 2010: 11). The task of the summit was to consolidate the field around 'practical strategies' for coping with this individualized conceptualization of pain.

The primary strategy endorsed by the summit's final report was a biopsychosocial model for dealing with pain (National Pain Summit Initiative 2010). Under the biopsychosocial model three key aspects of the patient are described as important, and they have been briefly summarized as "'Bio-' (what's happening to the body)… '-psycho-' (what's happening to the person)… [and] '-social' (what's happening in the person's world)" (Cohen and Wodak 2012: 24–25). It is important, however, to recognize that, while the biopsychosocial model is endorsed by the specialty of pain medicine, general medicine has not taken to the approach quite as readily. Cohen and Wodak note that:

> Although pain is appreciated conceptually in a 'biopsychosocial' framework that identifies semantic, psychological, societal and cultural contributions, the person in pain is still commonly processed through a narrow biomedical model, where the emphasis is on finding—and treating—an underlying pathological condition that 'causes' the pain. (2010: 10)

Tension between the biopsychosocial model and more conventional biomedical approaches is thought to contribute to the medical profession's stigmatization of the chronic pain patient (Morgan 2006: 38).

Despite this, pain medicine has maintained advocacy for the cautious use of opiates in the treatment of chronic pain. This has been the long-standing and largely consensus position of the specialty ever since an influential article on pain management by Portenoy and Foley in 1986: the article concludes that opiates are a 'safe, salutary and more humane alternative to the options of surgery or no treatment' (Portenoy and Foley 1986: 171). Continued advocacy for the use of opiates in the face of concern about their ability to be 'abused' often draws on neurological research about tolerance and dependence.

Tolerance, Dependence and 'Addiction'

As part of attempts to formulate a scientific literature to support a biopsychosocial model of pain and its treatment with opiate medications, pain medicine has drawn considerably from new neurological research. Since the early 1990s, a focus on the molecular and intracellular elements in neurological research has been presented as a 'cutting edge' way to demonstrate the 'plasticity' of the human brain. Though different areas of medicine and research have used the concept differently, 'neuroplasticity' and 'neuroadaptation' have been key explanatory tools for pain medicine. Drawing from the concept of neuroadaptation, pain medicine literature has built careful distinctions around the 'addictive' capacity of opiate medications. This section will outline neurological research about tolerance, dependence and 'opiate addiction', as well as the way pain medicine borrows from and interprets this research.

Neuroadaptation is described as 'the process by which the brain modifies its sensory input, in response to touch, heat, cold, pain, sight, sounds, or smell' (Kershner 2008: 302). In neurological research, the human brain is presented as having qualities of plasticity that render it susceptible to change in response to chemical stimulation (Hyman and Malenka 2001). The neuroplasticity of the brain forms one of the central tenets of neurological accounts of 'addiction' as a brain disease.

A wide range of scientific communities (Vrecko 2010) now advocate for a model of addiction as brain disease. This approach is primarily based on explanations of the neurobiological processes involved in drug use. Changes in the brain brought about by the chemical stimulation of prolonged opiate use are thus thought to produce the disease entity of 'addiction'. This is made visible, and ostensibly measurable, through a series of biomedical technologies such as positron emission tomography and functional magnetic resonance imaging (fMRI) scans that purport to show 'addiction' in particular color patterns, as contrasted with 'healthy' parts of the brain (Leshner 1997, 2001).

The US National Institute on Drug Abuse (NIDA) is a pioneer of the addiction as brain disease model and information on its website describes addiction as a "chronic, relapsing brain disease" brought about by the way in which "drugs change the brain; they change its structure and how it works" (2007). Neurological models specifically locate addiction in the malfunctioning of the pleasure-center of the brain. A distinction between 'normal' desire for the pleasurable effects of drugs and a 'disordered' pathological desire features prominently in the literature. There is, however, an unresolved tension in conceptualizing the brain as having properties of plasticity and thus as always subject to change, and the assumption that contact with opiates and other drugs creates a neurologically fixed disease state (addition). The literature only addresses these tensions by saying that addiction-related changes to the structure of the human brain present as particularly persistent (Fraser et al. 2014).

While addiction science presents 'drug addiction' as a neurobiological brain disease, its capacity to describe the way such neurological processes translate into specific social behaviors is limited. This demonstrates some of the tensions between addiction science and its translation into psychiatric diagnostic tools like the DSM-5. Addiction science seeks to provide an account of the causal relationship between drug use and the brain disease 'drug addiction', but fails to provide an explanation of how such neurological processes become complex human and social behaviors. There are also important tensions between what neurological accounts of tolerance represent in different areas of medicine. Though tolerance and withdrawal play less of a role in the DSM-5, they are still presented on a spectrum of mental disorder.

Pain medicine presents another account of the neurological process of tolerance due to prolonged opiate use. A basic consensus lies in the qualities of the neurological process of treating chronic pain with opiates, which is often described as such: "in the course of opioid treatment, the analgesic effects of opioids may show a decline with a given dose, or require a higher dose to produce an equivalent degree of analgesia" (Berger 2005: 113). This need to increase dosage of opiates is commonly presented as a 'red flag' in addiction discourse (Fraser et al. 2014). However, the pain medicine literature insists that an increase in dosage of opiates is normal and entirely manageable through appropriate clinical practice (Cohen and Wodak 2012). In such an account, the physiology of drug tolerance is rejected as an indication of addiction. Pain medicine has thus used the concept of neuroadaptation to, at least in part normalize drug tolerance in the context of the treatment of chronic pain (Rose 2003).

Within pain medicine, a series of terms have been developed to explain the neurological and behavioral consequences of prolonged opiate consumption among chronic pain patients. 'Pseudoaddiction' is used to describe drug-seeking behavior as a result of the under treatment of pain (Passik and Kirsh 2004). 'Therapeutic dependence' refers to similar behaviors produced by a patient's fear of running out of their prescription or of a worsening of their condition (Littlejohn et al. 2004). 'Chemical coping' is used to refer to a patient who (ab)uses their medications non-medically in order to deal with stress and anxiety related to chronic pain (Kwon et al. 2014). Thus, within the pain medicine literature 'true addiction' is "characterized by aberrant behavior, craving and loss of control", while prescription opiates are regarded as "not dangerous illicit substances but effective analgesics appropriate for long-term use" (Keane and Hamill 2010: 58). There are, however, noteworthy tensions between the pain medicine literature's attempt to avoid use of the term 'addiction' because of its stigmatizing qualities and the way in which chronic pain patients are stigmatized in medical practice (Cohen et al. 2011; Holloway et al. 2007; Jackson 2005).

The use of terms such as pseudoaddiction, therapeutic dependence and chemical coping also reifies long-standing distinctions between the psychical and psychological components of addiction. The physiological/psychological distinction developed by psychiatrists during the 1920s reappears, albeit in a slightly different form, in much of the pain medicine literature. As discussed in Chapter 2, the psychological/psychological distinction involves moral assumptions about people who have become dependent through 'legitimate' medical treatment and 'true addicts' who have become dependent through pleasure seeking. This literature also consolidates social distinctions between medical and criminal substances, licit and illicit opiates.

The distinctions between tolerance, dependence and 'addiction' presented by the pain medicine literature are held together by a faith in the medical profession and its role as an agent of social control. It is, however, worth noting that emerging concern about painkiller 'abuse' has somewhat challenged medicine's capacity for social control, leading to criticisms about a liberal prescribing culture around opiates (Kalso et al. 2010; Passik et al. 2011). Despite concerns about the liberal prescribing of opiates, the medical practitioner still retains a key social control element in much diagnostic practice. As noted in the previous chapter, the DSM-5 also upholds these distinctions by excluding tolerance and dependence as criteria for SUD if they present as part of treatment for chronic pain. Neurological research plays an important part in the changes made to the DMS-5. However, as this section has already indicated, there are a range of applications for neurological accounts of the plasticity of the human brain.

The Neuroscience of Pain

Neurological research has also been influential in other areas of pain medicine and research. The term neuroadaptation has also been used to refer to the way in which the experience of prolonged pain itself alters the functioning of the brain. Neurological research has helped build a scientific literature around the biopsychosocial model endorsed by pain medicine. Presenting psychological and social experiences as part of a process that alters the patient's brain provides a more recognizable medical narrative that returns to material and thus ostensibly measurable components of the body. However, pain medicine does not support any sort of consensus on the notion that neuroadaptive pain should be understood as pathological (Tracey and Bushnell 2009). Rather, much of the literature suggests that, much like drug tolerance, neurological changes to the brain as a result of pain is simply a normal neurological response to the experience of intense pain (Post 2002).

The neurological focus of the specialty has produced observations about the similarities of chronic pain, sustained opiate consumption and prolonged mood states such as depression and anxiety (Bair et al. 2008; Eisenberger 2012). Medical literature has long acknowledged a statistical association between chronic pain and the development of depression and anxiety (Fishbain et al. 1997). Similar observations have been made about physical and mental health more generally. A 2007 article in the Lancet on the global state of mental health states:

> The burden of mental disorders is likely to have been underestimated because of inadequate appreciation of the connectedness between mental illness and other health conditions. Because these interactions are protean, there can be no health without mental health. (Prince et al. 2007: 859)

The connection between mental and physical health is also associated with social status. In a report commissioned by the Government of the United Kingdom, the authors state:

> Mental health problems can also contribute to perpetuating cycles of inequality through generations... Many mental health problems start early and are associated with a number of known risk factors, including inequality. (HM Government 2011: 9–19)

Indeed, it is a consistent finding across an extensive breadth of research that social status (low levels of income, positioning within minority communities, etc.) is associated with a less robust physical condition as well as adverse psychological states (Teesson et al. 2011). While areas of medical and epidemiological research have demonstrated links between physical, psychological and social health outcomes, new neurological research has begun to note similarities in the neurological processes involved in physical, emotional and social forms of pain.

Neurological reports consistently find that social (which involves emotional) and physical pain share similar neurological mechanisms (MacDonald and Leary 2005). Neurological research has compared brain activity when exposed to physical injury and emotional anguish, finding noteworthy similarities. Studies using fMRI claim that 'certain human brain areas that 'light up' during physical pain are also activated during emotional pain induced by social exclusion' (Panksepp 2003: 237). A recent study extended observations using fMRI by testing the 'dorsal anterior cingulate cortex, anterior insula and operculum, and secondary somatosensory cortex and dorsal posterior insula individually', finding that "[e]ach region was activated by social pain" (Wager et al. 2013: 1395). Such neurological accounts have led researchers to posit that "social and physical pain might rely on overlapping neural processes in the form of a common neural alarm system" (Eisenberger and Lieberman 2004: 298). Within pain medicine literature neurological accounts of 'social pain' provide a biophysical explanation for statistical links between physical, emotional and social health. This aligns closely with the biopsychosocial approach and its focus on treating the biological, psychological and social factors of chronic pain as intimately related.

Neurological accounts of pain raise questions about the nature and experience of pain, which cannot be reduced to a simple matter of torn or damaged tissue. Specialized medical literature presents the experience of pain as an entirely subjectively experience. Widely accepted medical definitions of pain no longer require the verification of tissue damage and now include human experiences that are simply described in such terms. Developments in the neurological sciences have seen the principles of pain medicine extended to experiences of social exclusion and the emotional responses that accompany it. These developments reveal an expanded definition of pain in medical discourse and its approach to the health and illness of the human body. In order to better conceptualize the relationship between the physical, psychological and social elements of pain, the next section will canvass social science literature about the body.

The Body in the Social Sciences

The relationship between the physical body and the social world has often been the subject of social science research and scholarship. Such research has demonstrated how social forces shape cultural understandings of the body. This section will outline social science literature about the medical perspective and the way it constructs the body, illness and pain.

In Foucault's work around the genealogy of the medical perspective, he notes that its development in the eighteenth century relied on a construction of the body as either functional or dysfunctional (1994). The identification of disease (or ill-health more broadly) relies on medicine's generalized understanding of what is 'normal' bodily functioning. Any deviation from this understanding of normative bodily function could then be reduced to a pathological classification (Foucault 1994). Describing acute pain as an indicator of injury or illness has important links to this traditional medical view of the body and continues to inform general medicine's ongoing commitment to biomedical (as opposed to biopsychosocial) understandings of the patient, the body and pain.

Sociological interest in the body since the 1960s has built on Foucault's (1994) observation that twentieth-century medical practice involved increased surveillance of the body, through the institutionalization of routine medical examinations and the establishment of the postmortem and surgical fields. This work introduced a theoretical framework that presented the body to be the 'ultimate site of political and ideological control, surveillance and regulation… thus rendering bodies productive and politically and economically useful' (Lupton 2012: 25).

Due in part to a desire to avoid a biological deterministic perspective, the social sciences have long been reluctant to directly engage the body as a site of scholarly interest (Turner 1984). There are, however, traditions of sociology that have long been interested in the medical profession and the way it understands health and illness. The functionalist tradition of the sociology of health and illness established that the identification of disease and illness is a bureaucratic (Strong 1979) and social process (Parsons 1951), while Marxist traditions have emphasized the impacts of the inequalities produced by the capitalist economic system (Conrad and Schneider 1980; Illich 1976).

In 1984, Turner's influential *The Body and Society* established a foundation for, what came to be known as, the sociology of the body. Turner elaborated on an understanding that the body (and its illness) is the subject of power relations: 'The language of disease involves judgment as to what is desirable and undesirable, and the medical profession has in modern society enormous institutional purchase on what is to count as the good life' (Turner 1984: 200). The role of the patient in 'confessing' the diseased or unwell body is an important element of the sociological literature (Armstrong 1983), and particularly resonant for interpretations of medical approaches to pain. It was in 1979 that the IASP created its definition of pain as a subjectively verifiable phenomenon within the medical clinic. The ambiguous relationship between the materiality of pain and representations of pain also haunts medicine's inability to arrive at a satisfactory tool of 'measurement'.

Scarry's seminal piece on torture, *The Body in Pain (1985)*, noted that unlike other bodily experiences pain has no external object: 'Hearing and touch are of objects outside the boundaries of the body, as desire is desire of x, fear is fear of y, hunger is hunger for z; but pain is not 'of' or 'for' anything – it is itself alone' (1985: 161–162). The absence of an external object makes pain unique from other human experiences, because it often defies expression, whether in individual or medical discourse. The struggle to find meaning in and proper expression for pain has since been the subject of critical theory (Morris 1991), sociological inquiry (Illouz 2013) and anthropological study (Good et al. 1994).

In an investigation into the "uncertain geographies of pain" Bissel describes the multiple possible elements of material expressions of pain:

> First, there is the affective force of the physical painfulness of the pain itself impressing through the body: the sheer bite of pain through the body itself... Indeed this might be supplemented by the communication of the 'bite' of pain through facial expressions and bodily comportments. But then there is the affect of the hospital that intensifies the embodied sensation of the physical pain, the clenched fists, the thumping of the heart, through its proximity. (Bissel 2012: 81)

Bissel's account describes the way the body communicates pain, and the way representational systems ascribed to such expression also inform the experience of pain.

The emergence of social constructionist accounts of the body since the 1980s has also illustrated that, while the body contains certain fixed capacities (such as height and bone structure), the body is also mediated by "certain kinds of knowledge and discourses which are subject to change" (Lupton 2012: 23). The contributions of the sociology of health and illness, as well as the emergence of the sociology of the body, have helped to remake cultural understandings of the body. Social science research has demonstrated that there is an intimate relationship between the body and the social world. The way the body is governed is thus also an important area of social science literature on the body.

The governmentality literature has noted that since the 1980s medical and public health discourses have increasingly 'emphasized [that] the mundane striving for "good" or "perfect" health involves intensive 'work on the self' or self-governance' (Petersen et al. 2010: 392). Castel's work in the influential *The Foucault Effect* (1991) noted an important transition in neoliberal societies from forms of social control based on 'face-to-face' relationships with experts to those based on abstracted calculations of risk. Petersen has extended these observations by noting that neoliberal modes of public health erode the distinction between sickness and health, replacing it with an "endless parade of 'at risk' populations and 'risky' situations" (1997: 195). Elements of public health have encouraged individuals to 'take responsibility' for the condition of the body, including the pain it is subject to, by negotiating risks to their health (Petersen and Lupton 1996).

A language of 'empowerment' plays an important role in this neoliberal philosophy about health. Yet for most self-governance of the body through the responsible management of risk appears as an elite ideal that is unachievable without considerable financial resources. The governmentality field has developed a distinct skepticism of the notion that neoliberal approaches to public health provide any sort of genuine tool of a-political 'empowerment': 'despite the language of empowerment and freedom, this striving for health entails compulsion, added responsibilities to others, and often punishment and social exclusion in the case of those who fail to conform' (Petersen et al. 2010: 392).

Applications of governmentality have produced a substantive body of scholarship politicizing the neoliberal fantasy of 'empowering individuals' through 'government at a distance'. As well as outlining the responsibilization of health practice (Gray 2009; Teghtsoonian 2009), this literature has also demonstrates how neoliberal governance has been used to justify a retreat from the 'welfare state', seen most clearly through the privatization of health and social services (Blomqvist 2013; Larner 2000). Governmentality scholars have used 'technologies of self' as a way to explain the imposition of prevailing health discourse that demands the production of a more enterprising subject, in charge of his/her own health.

However, much of this literature has been critiqued for providing a limited analysis of neoliberal governance, one that reproduces a top-down model of power by readily privileging 'official' discourses (O'Malley et al. 1997) and thus discounting the constitutive role of resistance in Foucault's original account of governmentality (Mckee 2009). In the analysis of the governance of bodies and pain, a balance needs to be struck between examination of wider social structures and the individual body being governed. The remainder of the chapter will address the biopolitical arrangements that shape and impact the body in pain.

Anxious Bodies, Anxious Selves

Due in part to the ways in which bodies are governed in late-modern society, definitions of pain have been extended to include feelings of 'anxiety'. Medical accounts of pain often incorporate notions of anxiety. Pain medicine literature includes explanations of pain patients who feel anxious about a worsening of their condition and who engage in anxious 'drug seeking' (Kirsh et al. 2007). The neurological literature often refers to 'anxious attachments' and their contribution to forms of social pain (Eisenberger 2011). A range of pharmacotherapies, largely framed under a psychological paradigm, have also been developed over the last century to deal with a growing emphasis on anxiety.

However, it is important to remember that a history of medical intervention into pain and its connection to anxiety may disguise the social determinants of 'feeling worried'. It is thus also necessary to consider the way social theorists have described the uncertain conditions of modernity, and how this contributes to people's bodily experiences of pain. The conditions of modern society shape the production of affective states and the manner in which they are experienced, labeled, understood and responded to individually and socially. This section articulates how the 'age of anxiety' described in Chapter 1 intersects with medical accounts of anxiety disorders and the way they are treated and understood as the alleviation of pain or suffering.

The fragmentation of late-modern societies articulated by social theorists such as Bauman (2007) and Beck et al. (1994) highlights the way conditions of uncertainty are ever-present in the contemporary world. Not only are modernist institutions less stable and less reliable in the contemporary world, but capitalism has also adapted to profit from the notion of individualized self-discipline that have emerged to fill the gap they left. Neoliberal capitalism plays on uncertainty about social identity and structure, courting the anxieties of the consumer to convince them to consume any number of products that will 'keep the doctor away' (Salecl 2004). Healthy living through changes to diet, exercise and 'lifestyle' is a staple of the modern-day middle class and those who aspire to it. Failure to live up to the ideal flexible subject, who is entrepreneurial in their career and self-disciplined in managing the health of their body, is met with social exclusion or moral distain (Petersen et al. 2010). Such changes in modern society may indeed be fostering uncertainty and thus produce social and emotional 'worry' that is likely to be experienced and understood as painful.

There are noticeable similarities between observations in social theory and notions of dispersed neoliberal governance outlined in the previous section. These elaborations of modernity describe an uncertain and unpredictable time that may itself produce feelings of anxiety divorced of any pathological origin. Still, it is important to account for the ways in which anxiety has been produced as a bodily experience that is often read as a form of dysfunction.

The language of stress and the introduction of 'mood medicine' are examples of the prominent role of pain metaphors in articulating the subjective experience and impacts of the conditions of late-modernity. The work of endocrinologist Hans Selye in the 1930s was the first to produce a scientific account of 'stress'. Though Selye's work used 'stress' as a way to describe the body's response to external stimuli (1950), processes of medicalization shifted the meaning of the term to refer to the external stimuli itself (1977). Stress quickly came to represent circumstances outside of people's control that made them psychologically uneasy (Dowbiggin 2009). Physicians soon became interested in medicine's ability to manage or alleviate this kind of distress. The emergence of, what has been termed 'mood medicine' developed alongside the introduction of tranquilizers into the pharmaceutical repertoire available in the 1950s. Dubbed 'happy pills' and 'emotional aspirin' the use of tranquilizers gave the impression that medicine could manage and control people's responses to stress (Speaker 1997).

The related terminology of anxiety became increasingly common after the end of the Second World War, especially as it was applied to returning war veterans. Stress-related anxiety, panic and social phobia became integrated into the diagnostic criteria of a broad range of psychological conditions. By 1980, in the third edition of the DSM, anxiety-related panic and social phobia became stand-alone categories of psychological diagnosis. As the first drugs approved for the treatment of panic disorder (among other psychological diagnosis), alprazolam (marketed as Xanax®), and later fluoxetine (marketed as Prozac® in the US and Lovan® in Australia) were introduced in the 1980s. The introduction of paroxetine (Seroxat® and Paxil®) for the treatment of social phobia followed in the 1990s (Lexchin 2001). As is emblematic of medical practice, the increased availability and popularity of these medications accelerated a process of legitimizing the disorders they purported to treat (Shorter and Marshall 1997).

By the twenty-first century, a long history of pathologizing stress and anxiety (briefly summarized above) provided socially acceptable and medically legitimate ways of understanding and interpreting the physical sensations that accompany emotional uncertainty: 'People who feel the aches, pains, and up-and-down emotions of everyday life soon learn that these symptoms have a medical name, which makes them all the more sensitive to their bodily sensations' (Dowbiggin 2009: 434). Anxious concern about job insecurity, social awkwardness or healthy living in late-modernity may also produce the 'facial expressions and bodily comportments' (2012: 81) that Bissel described earlier as specific to embodied encounters with physical pain. Crying, clench fists and a thumping heart are not bodily responses specific to physical injury, as social and emotional worry may also elicit a similar response.

Anxiety about the body and forms of emotional distress also extend to other areas of medical intervention and the commercial sphere. Poststructuralist traditions of sociology have even argued that, in contemporary society anxieties about the body are conflated with anxieties about the self. Following Turner's articulation of a sociology of the body, during the 1980s Featherstone began writing about the modification of the body as a process of inscribing selfhood. Taking consumption as an important frame, Featherstone articulates a context of individualized consumption in which people are encouraged to alter their bodies through consumption, and in doing so stake a claim over who they are:

> [T]he tendency within consumer culture is for ascribed bodily qualities to become regarded as plastic – with effort and 'body work' individuals are persuaded that they can achieve a certain desired appearance. (Featherstone 1982: 22)

Poststructuralists note that in consumer discourse consumption is presented as an important political act. The ability to consume is equated with the ability to express oneself.

The ability to fully express oneself and its apparent link to consumption is murkier when applied to the area of social interaction. Medical interventions into social and emotional problems often come up against questions about the way pharmaceuticals can alter selfhood. The controversy that surrounded rising interest in and a backlash against the effects of Prozac during the 1980s provides a good illustration of the vagaries of medicating emotions. Kramer, an American Psychiatrist, authored a book about his experiences with the prescription of Prozac during the 1980s, in which he discusses a client named Tess:

> I prescribed [Prozac] for Tess, for entirely conventional reasons – to ameliorate her depression more thoroughly, to return to her 'premorbid self'... But medications do not always behave as we expect them to. (1994: 7)

Kramer goes on to write that at his next appointment with Tess he observed a significant transformation in her intimate, social and professional relationships:

> It makes a psychiatrist uneasy to watch a medicated patient change her circle of friends, her demeanor at work, her relationship to her family… To ameliorate depression is all very well, but it was less clear how psychiatrists were to use a medication that could lend social ease, command, even brilliance… And always there was the question of how society would be affected by our access to drugs that alter personality in desirable ways. (1994: 12)

Indeed, it is significant that Tess reports that her newfound confidence did not last once she ceased use of the drug. After going 8 months without Prozac Tess returned to Kramer saying "she was slipping":

> 'I am not myself.' But who had she been all those years if not herself? Had medication somehow removed a false self and replaced it with a true one? Might Tess, absent the invention of the modern antidepressant, have lived her whole life… and never been herself. (1994: 19)

Tess' example illustrates the blurred intersections of broadened understandings of pain relief and the modification of selfhood implied through forms of medication consumption (Wolf 2002).

Similar debates have surrounded the prescription of methylphenidate (Ritalin) as pharmacotherapy for attention deficit hyperactivity disorder (ADHD). Social theorists have questioned this mode of 'treating' ADHD based on people, and mainly children's ability to 'fit in', implying that it may disguise processes of social engineering (Conrad and Potter 2000; Searight and McLaren 1998). Use of paroxetine (Seroxat® and Paxil®) has also been criticized for pathologizing 'shyness' through the treatment of 'social phobia':

> [In 2000] SmithKline Beecham received approval to market paroxetine for the treatment of social phobia as defined by the Diagnostic and Statistical Manual of Mental Disorders. This disorder can be distressing and disabling for those who suffer from it, limiting their ability to

> interact with the outside world. But what we now risk, given the cultural acceptance of (and perhaps preference for) an extrovert norm, is an extension of the definition of social phobia to include shyness: a normal character trait of some people who have no psychiatric disease is turned into an abnormality that requires treatment. (Lexchin 2001: 1449)

Recent incarnations of the debate about pharmacotherapy for 'erectile dysfunction' are also of note (Kim and Uhl 2011). Critical accounts of use of the drug have argued that, through its presentation as a biomedical problem, 'erectile dysfunction' becomes disconnected from the social and cultural expectations about masculinity and sexuality that constitute it to be problematic (Johnson and Åsberg 2012).

In Carl Elliott's influential book *Better Than Well* (2004), the author ponders American society's growing embrace of 'enhancement technologies'. Elliot's work explores confronting ethical questions posed by medical technologies that consciously act to 'enhance' rather than 'cure', often with important consequences on notions of selfhood. Aspects of Elliot's work are inspired by the manufacture of a series of, what were subsequently termed 'lifestyle drugs' during the 1990s (Williams et al. 2009). Elliot was particularly skeptical of the prescription of antidepressants and stimulants, which he argues contain the capacity to alter the self in socially amenable ways. This is not to deny the suffering that accompanies the conditions for which these medications are prescribed. However, to reduce anxiety, depression, ADHD, social phobia, and erectile dysfunction to biomedical frameworks ignores the ways in which they are socially constructed around ideals of the good life, productive citizenship, extrovert personality and gender norms.

Within late-modern societies an inability to fully express yourself, within established social norms, is increasingly experienced as a form of suffering. Feelings of anxiety are reduced to a pathological classification that locates them in the individual. The way in which pharmacotherapies, like alprazolam, fluoxetine, methylphenidate and paroxetine, alter the physiology of the body also has important consequences on people's sense of self. These kinds of approaches to pain do not, however, simply emerge organically; they have arisen alongside the encroachment of commercial interests into the medical perspective.

The Commercialization of Pain

The notion of the body-as-self has also been taken up by commercial interests seeking to capitalize on expanded understandings of pain. Examples of the encroachment of commercial interests in the construction and alleviation of pain have already been alluded to throughout the chapter. Salecl (2004) noted how advanced liberal economies rely on the reproduction of the anxieties of the modern consumer. Social anxieties about notions of ideal extrovert personality are likely to be feeding the genuine suffering of people who feel alienated by an inability to interact in social settings. The potential to profit from pharmaceutical intervention into the lives of people who do not meet the ideals of modern citizenship requires close scrutiny.

The commercialization of pain also has notable connections to neoliberal trends in public health. Aspects of public health discourse and policy assume 'White' and middle-class ideals about the accessibility and actionably of knowledge about heath. One of the consequences of this approach has been the development of a discourse of self-care in aspects of public health rhetoric. Self-care rhetoric is particularly evident in the way contemporary public health has recently embraced digital technology as a way of apparently 'empowering' the patient (Greene and Hibbard 2012). Lupton has noted that the introduction of 'digitalised health information systems, the employment of wireless mobile digital devices and wearable, implanted or inserted biosensors' has encouraged an understanding of 'lay persons' as a '"participant" who is actively involved in self-care' (Lupton 2013: 258). Of course, access to such technology often involves significant costs. People's ability to be 'empowered' by these technologies is thus proportional to the financial resources available to them.

Technological advancements such as the internet are often presented as more democratic in their ability to empower people to engage in self-care. The Australian Self Medication Industry (ASMI) association is an organization largely funded by the pharmaceutical industry to advocate for direct-to-consumer access—or access without medical prescriptions—for a greater number of medications. Originally established in 1974, the ASMI encourages "Better Health Through Responsible Self Care" (2014). Promotional material on ASMIs website explains a shift in the association's focus toward 'self-care' since 2000 as such:

> The take-up of Self Care coincides with a growing interest in personal health and wellbeing, increased access to a wide range of health information… The idea that individuals should take greater responsibility for their health also fits with a growing trend of consumer empowerment. (2014)

The association's explicit stated purpose is to provide 'A roadmap towards greater personal responsibility in managing health'. The website provides a range of information that purports to help consumers make choices about forms of self-care. These kinds of tools are presented as key to the dissemination of health knowledge and thus allow for the apparent empowerment of the modern health consumer. Commercial interest in allowing consumers to gain direct access to medications is thus disguised in neoliberal rhetoric about self-care.

There are, however, more subtle examples of the commercial interests involved in a neoliberal push for self-care. The Victorian Government produces a website called the Better Health Channel in which research and information about health are disseminated to a broad audience. On the site's Wellbeing page, it states 'Wellbeing is not just the absence of disease or illness. It is a complex combination of a person's physical, mental, emotional and social health factors' (State Government of Victoria 2013). The site also indicates that 'researchers investigating happiness' have identified the following factors that influence wellbeing:

> Happy intimate relationship with a partner, network of close friends, enjoyable and fulfilling career, enough money, regular exercise, nutritional diet, sufficient sleep, spiritual or religious beliefs, fun hobbies and leisure pursuits, healthy self-esteem, optimistic outlook, realistic and achievable goals, sense of purpose and meaning, a sense of belonging, the ability to adapt to change and living in a fair and democratic society. (State Government of Victoria 2013)

Information about government services that might deliver these "physical, mental, emotional and social health factors" is, however, noticeably absent. Instead, the website acts largely as a summary of the broad cross section of information about how to achieve a state of conflated health/happiness—its implicit purpose seems be a tool to encourage a kind of informed self-discipline. Such websites do little more than provide health information, yet may be presented as apparent alternatives to traditional health and social services.

As part of a broader reconceptualization of health at an international level, medical and health discourse is no longer focused simply on correcting dysfunctional bodies (World Health Organization 2014). The State Government of Victoria boasts an entire website dedicated to optimizing the health, and thus happiness of its citizens. Commercial interests have sought to capitalize on this expansion of the parameters of health (and medicine), by seeking to shift the onus of achieving it onto to the lay consumer. Industry groups such as ASMI actively lobby for these kinds of expansions to the parameters of self-care.

There are also significant appropriations of the concepts discussed thus far in the current landscape of direct-to-consumer advertisements for pain medications. A wide range of advertisements for over-the-counter analgesic medications draw on the notion that physical pain inhibits the body, and by extension the self. The physical anguish felt by pain is supplemented by the way it denies or suspends the individual's ability to participate in contemporary society. Within the commercial space, pain is described as an interrupting force on the body, that necessarily cripples or compromises the self. Consumption is thus presented as an important method of remediating, and perhaps even enhancing the body-as-self.

A recent Panadol® advertisement declares, 'Life happens fast. Don't miss out' (2012), while another insists that 'There's never a good time to have a headache' (2012). Whether it be on your wedding day, during a workout, or in the middle of an action packed espionage mission, the physical presence of headache pain is presented as an interrupting force that detracts from modern life (Reckitt Benckiser (Australia) Pty Limited 2010). One advertisement for Nurofen® tablets shows a range of people with visible signs of discomfort from headache pain that interrupts their ability to go surfing, take a ballet class, go jogging, take care of the kids, work productively in the office and study in the library. According to the advertisement, the answer is of course to take two Nurofen tablets, which appear brightly lit in the final shot.

In an international television advertisement for Panadol Extra® a man is shown sitting, leant over, with hands on head, while animated ripples of a threatening shade of red radiate across his body. The narrator says "If tough pain gets in the way try new Panadol Extra Advanced®" (visit4ads 2012). As the narrator lists the apparent advantages of the new product, the animated ripples of red 'pain' dissipate and the male figure is freed to flip off a dive board and energetically cut through the water of a lap pool.

These kinds of advertisements depict a wide range of people engaging in a wide range of social activities. They draw on social anxieties about child rearing, healthy living and productive work, with over-the-counter analgesics presented as the answer to those anxieties. Pain medications are thus presented as drugs that manage the consumer's ability to participate in leisure activities, child rearing and productive work and/or study—mention of analgesia is rare and only ever peripheral. In advertisements for over-the-counter pain medications pain relief is not simply about alleviating physical discomfort, it also incorporates a significant component of being able to 'live life to the fullest'. The line between pain relief and self-enhancement becomes blurred and indistinct. Thus, the ability to 'live life to the fullest' is placed in the hands of the consumer, who simply needs to buy and consume painkillers in order to get on with the day. Taking care of the self is presented as a matter of consumption: the suggestion is that if you consume the right products you will be pain free, live life to fullest and perhaps even enhance the self.

Conclusion

This chapter has explored medical, social and commercial approaches to pain. It has revealed tensions from within the medical perspective and its implications for the consumption of pain medications. Given that the diagnosis of pain relies almost solely on the patient's perspective, chronic pain in particular delivers a potent challenge to the standard empowerment of the medical expert in the doctor/patient relationship (Baszanger 1992). Pain medicine and its emphasis on individualized experiences of pain have thus necessarily expanded the definition of what it is to be in pain beyond the parameters of physical discomfort.

As understandings of pain have expanded, the expectation that the body can be free from pain also translates to an expectation that the self can be cured of social anxiety and emotional unrest. In a social context that assumes that the body can be medically controlled, medication consumers anticipate an increased capacity for medical technologies to alleviate suffering. However, as the specialty of pain medicine has emphasized, pain relief is not always a priority in the medical profession. Partly informed by physicians concerned about being accused of 'pedaling' a 'drug of abuse', there is no identifiable drive in the medical profession to make pain medications more broadly available. The regulation and consumption of painkillers are thus characterized by a tension between the medical promise to alleviate pain and the professional and institutional limitations placed on that promise.

Developments in the sociology of health and illness, and related interests in anthropology and cultural studies, help to articulate shifts in and current understandings of the body in pain. No longer simply represented as an indicator of bodily malfunction, the experience of pain invites a series of complex questions about sociality and selfhood. What does it mean to describe emotions and anxieties that may be socially produced under medical frameworks that have pharmaceutical solutions? How are people expected to distinguish between consumption for pain relief and consumption for self-enhancement? These questions remain unanswered in the medical literature.

One response to the tensions in the medical perspective and the expansion of pain to include social and emotional forms of suffering has been a deferral to the neoliberal subject: who is encouraged to find individualized ways to manage the kind of uncertainty and fluidity that characterizes late-modern society. Neoliberal discourse and the commercial interests that accompany it have sought to capitalize on these broadened understandings of pain. Contemporary approaches to the body as the location of the self, and which is subject to change through commercial consumption, have important implications on the way pain is labeled, experienced and treated.

In the context outlined here, people's individualized appropriation of medical discourse and practice may well provide a compelling alternative to the psychopharmacological perspectives that have dominated much of the current research literature about non-medical consumption. The next part of the book will address some of the questions raised here by directly engaging the perspectives of those who themselves use painkillers non-medically.

References

Armstrong, D. (1983). *Political Anatomy of the Body: Medical Knowledge in Britain in the Twentieth Century*. Cambridge: Cambridge University Press.

Australian Self Medication Industry. (2014). *What Is Self Care?* Retrieved April 21, 2014, from http://www.asmi.com.au/self-care/What-Is-Self-Care.aspx.

Bair, M. J., Wu, J., Damush, T. M., Sutherland, J. M., & Kroenke, K. (2008). Association of Depression and Anxiety Alone and in Combination with Chronic Musculoskeletal Pain in Primary Care Patients. *Psychosomatic Medicine, 70*(8), 890–897.

Baszanger, I. (1992). Deciphering Chronic Pain. *Sociology of Health & Illness, 14*(2), 181–215.

Bauman, Z. (2007). *Liquid Times: Living in an Age of Uncertainty*. Cambridge: Wiley.

Beck, U., Giddens, A., & Lash, S. (1994). *Reflexive Modernization: Politics Tradition and Aesthetics in the Modern Social Order*. Stanford: Stanford University Press.

Berger, J. M. (2005). Opioids in Anesthesia. *Seminars in Anesthesia, Perioperative Medicine and Pain, 24*(2), 108–119.

Bissel, D. (2012). Placing Affective Relations: Uncertain Geographies of Pain. In P. Harrison & B. Anderson (Eds.), *Taking-Place: Non-Representational Theories and Geography*. Farnham: Ashgate.

Blomqvist, P. (2013). Citizenship, Choice and Social Equity in Welfare Services. In K. S. Helgesson & U. Mörth (Eds.), *The Political Role of Corporate Citizens: An Interdisciplinary Approach*. Basingstoke: Palgrave Macmillan.

Briggs, M., & Closs, J. S. (1999). A Descriptive Study of the Use of Visual Analogue Scales and Verbal Rating Scales for the Assessment of Postoperative Pain in Orthopedic Patients. *Journal of Pain and Symptom Management, 18*(6), 438–446.

Chapman, C. R., Casey, K. L., Dubner, R., Foley, K. M., Gracely, R. H., & Reading, A. E. (1985). Pain Measurement: An Overview. *Pain, 22*(1), 1–31.

Clark, N. (2010). Injectable Diacetylmorphine Is More Effective Than Oral Methadone in the Treatment of Chronic Relapsing Opioid Dependence. *Evidence Based Mental Health, 13*(3), 80–80.

Cohen, M., Quintner, J., Buchanan, D., Nielsen, M., & Guy, L. (2011). Stigmatization of Patients with Chronic Pain: The Extinction of Empathy. *Pain Medicine, 12,* 1637–1643.

Cohen, M. L., & Wodak, A. D. (2010). The Judicious Use of Opioids in Managing Chronic Noncancer Pain. *Medicine Today, 11*(2), 10–18.

Cohen, M. L., & Wodak, A. D. (2012). Opioid Prescribing in General Practice: A Proposed Approach. *Medicine Today, 13*(1), 24–32.

Conrad, P., & Potter, D. (2000). From Hyperactive Children to ADHD Adults: Observations on the Expansion on Medical Categories. *Social Problems, 47*(4), 559–582.

Conrad, P., & Schneider, J. W. (1980). *Deviance and Medicalization: From Badness to Sickness*. Philadelphia: Temple University Press.

Dallenbach, K. M. (1939). Pain: History and Present Status. *The American Journal of Psychology, 52*(3), 331–347.

Dowbiggin, I. R. (2009). High Anxieties: The Social Construction of Anxiety Disorders. *Canadian Journal of Psychiatry, 54*(7), 429–436.

Eisenberger, N. I. (2011). The Neural Basis of Social Pain: Findings and Implications. In G. MacDonald & L. A. Jensen-Campbell (Eds.), *Social Pain: Neuropsychological and Health Implications of Loss and Exclusion* (pp. 53–78). Washington: American Psychological Association.

Eisenberger, N. I. (2012). The Pain of Social Disconnection: Examining the Shared Neural Underpinnings of Physical and Social Pain. *Nature Reviews Neuroscience, 13*(6), 421–434.

Eisenberger, N. I., & Lieberman, M. D. (2004). Why Rejection Hurts: A Common Neural Alarm System for Physical and Social Pain. *Trends in Cognitive Sciences, 8*(7), 294–300.

Elliott, C., & Kramer, P. D. (2004). *Better Than Well: American Medicine Meets the American Dream*. New York: W. W. Norton & Company.

Featherstone, M. (1982). The Body in Consumer Culture. *Theory, Culture & Society, 1*(2), 18–33.
Ferrell, B. A. (2003). Acute and Chronic Pain. In C. K. Cassel (Eds.), *Geriatric Medicine: An Evidence-Based Approach*. New York: Springer.
Fishbain, D. A., Cutler, R., Rosomoff, H. L., & Rosomoff, R. S. (1997). Chronic Pain-Associated Depression: Antecedent or Consequence of Chronic Pain? A Review. *Clinical Journal of Pain, 13*(2), 116–137.
Foucault, M. (1991). *The Foucault Effect: Studies in Governmentality*. G. Burchell, C. Gordon, & P. Miller (Eds.). Chicago: University of Chicago Press.
Foucault, M. (1994). *The Birth of the Clinic: An Archaeology of Medical Perception* (A. Sheridan, Trans.). New York: Vintage Books.
Frampton, C. L., & Hughes-Webb, P. (2011). The Measurement of Pain. *Clinical Oncology, 23*(6), 381–386.
Fraser, S. (2008). Trauma, Damage and Pleasure: Rethinking Problematic Drug Use. *International Journal of Drug Policy, 19*(5), 410–416.
Fraser, S., Moore, D., & Keane, H. (2014). *Habits: Remaking Addiction*. Basingstoke: Palgrave Macmillan.
Good, M. J. D. V., Brodwin, P. E., Good, B. J., & Kleinman, A. (1994). *Pain as Human Experience: An Anthropological Perspective*. Berkeley and Los Angeles: University of California Press.
Gray, G. C. (2009). The Responsibilization Strategy of Health and Safety Neo-Liberalism and the Reconfiguration of Individual Responsibility for Risk. *British Journal of Criminology, 49*(3), 326–342.
Greene, J., & Hibbard, J. H. (2012). Why Does Patient Activation Matter? An Examination of the Relationships Between Patient Activation and Health-Related Outcomes. *Journal of General Internal Medicine, 27*(5), 520–526.
HM Government. (2011). *No Health Without Mental Health: A Cross-Government Mental Health Outcomes Strategy for People of All Ages*. London: HM Government.
Holloway, I., Sofaer-Bennett, B., & Walker, J. (2007). The Stigmatisation of People with Chronic Back Pain. *Disability and Rehabilitation, 29*(18), 1456–1464.
Hyman, S. E., & Malenka, R. C. (2001). Addiction and the Brain: The Neurobiology of Compulsion and Its Persistence. *Nature Reviews Neuroscience, 2*(10), 695–703.
Illich, I. (1976). *Medical Nemesis: The Expropriation of Health*. New York: Pantheon Books.

Illouz, E. (2013). *Why Love Hurts: A Sociological Explanation*. Oxford: Wiley.
International Association for the Study of Pain. (2014). *IASP Taxonomy.* Retrieved March 29, 2014, from https://www.iasp-pain.org/Education/Content.aspx?ItemNumber=1698.
Jackson, J. E. (2005). Stigma, Liminality, and Chronic Pain: Mind-Body Borderlands. *American Ethnologist, 32*(3), 332–353.
Johnson, E., & Åsberg, C. (2012). Enrolling Men, Their Doctors, and Partners: Individual and Collective Responses to Erectile Dysfunction. *Science & Technology Studies, 25*(2), 46–60.
Kalso, E., Hearn, L., & de Williams, A. C. (2010). Reducing the Risk of Opioid Misuse in Persistent Pain: Commentary on Jamison et al. *Pain, 150*(3), 375–376.
Keane, H., & Hamill, K. (2010). Variations in Addiction: The Molecular and the Molar in Neuroscience and Pain Medicine. *BioSocieties, 5*(1), 52–69.
Kershner, R. M. (2008). *Neuroadaptation and Multifocal IOLs: The Art of Science*. Thorofare: Slack.
Kim, M., & Uhl, K. (2011). Sex and Lifestyle Drugs: The Pursuit of the Fountain of Youth. *Clinical Pharmacology and Therapeutics, 89*(1), 3–9.
Kirsh, K. L., Jass, C., Bennett, D. S., Hagen, J. E., & Passik, S. D. (2007). Initial Development of a Survey Tool to Detect Issues of Chemical Coping in Chronic Pain Patients. *Palliative and Supportive Care, 5*(3), 219–226.
Kramer, P. D. (1994). *Listening to Prozac*. London: Penguin Books.
Kwon, J. H., Tanco, K., Hui, D., Reddy, A., & Bruera, E. (2014). Chemical Coping Versus Pseudoaddiction in Patients with Cancer Pain. *Palliative and Supportive Care, 12*(5), 413–417.
Larner, W. (2000). Neo-Liberalism: Policy, Ideology, Governmentality. *Studies in Political Economy, 63,* 5–25.
Leshner, A. I. (1997). Addiction Is a Brain Disease, and It Matters. *Science, 278*(5335), 45–47.
Leshner, A. (2001). Addiction Is a Brain Disease. *Issues in Science and Technology, 17*(2), 75–80.
Lexchin, J. (2001). Lifestyle Drugs: Issues for Debate. *Canadian Medical Association Journal, 164*(10), 1449–1451.
Littlejohn, C., Baldacchino, A., & Bannister, J. (2004). Chronic Non-Cancer Pain and Opioid Dependence. *Journal of the Royal Society of Medicine, 97*(2), 62–65.
Lupton, D. (2012). *Medicine as Culture: Illness, Disease and the Body*. London: Sage.

Lupton, D. (2013). The Digitally Engaged Patient: Self-Monitoring and Self-Care in the Digital Health Era. *Social Theory & Health, 11*(3), 256–270.
MacDonald, G., & Leary, M. R. (2005). Why Does Social Exclusion Hurt? The Relationship Between Social and Physical Pain. *Psychological Bulletin, 131*(2), 202–223.
Mckee, K. (2009). Post-Foucauldian Governmentality: What Does It Offer Critical Social Policy Analysis? *Critical Social Policy, 29*(3), 465–486.
Meldrum, M. L. (2003). A Capsule History of Pain Management. *Journal of the American Medical Association, 290*(18), 2470–2475.
Melzack, R. (1975). The McGill Pain Questionnaire: Major Properties and Scoring Methods. *Pain, 1*(3), 277–299.
Melzack, R. (1996). *Gate Control Theory: On the Evolution of Pain Concepts.* Paper Presented at the Pain Forum.
Melzack, R., & Wall, P. D. (1967). Pain Mechanisms: A New Theory. *Survey of Anesthesiology, 11*(2), 89–90.
Morgan, B. D. (2006). Knowing How to Play the Game: Hospitalized Substance Abusers' Strategies for Obtaining Pain Relief. *Pain Management Nursing, 7*(1), 31–41.
Morris, D. B. (1991). *The Culture of Pain.* Berkeley: University of California Press.
National Institute on Drug Abuse. (2007). *Drugs, Brain and Behaviour: The Science of Addiction.* Retrieved January 13, 2012, from http://www.drugabuse.gov/sites/default/files/sciofaddiction.pdf.
National Pain Summit Initiative. (2010). *National Pain Strategy: Pain Management for All Australians.* Sydney: MBF Foundation & University of Sydney Pain Management Research Institute.
Noble, B., Clark, D., Meldrum, M., Have, H. T., Seymour, J., Winslow, M., et al. (2005). The Measurement of Pain, 1945–2000. *Journal of Pain and Symptom Management, 29*(1), 14–21.
Northern Private Pain Centre. (2012). *What Is Chronic Pain?* Retrieved January 22, 2014, from http://www.northernpaincentre.com.au/what-is-chronic-pain/w1/i1001394/.
Nosyk, B., Guh, D. P., Bansback, N. J., Oviedo-Joekes, E., Brissette, S., Marsh, D. C., Meikleham, E., Schechter, M. T., & Anis, A. H. (2012). Cost-Effectiveness of Diacetylmorphine Versus Methadone for Chronic Opioid Dependence Refractory to Treatment. *Canadian Medical Association Journal, 184*(6), E317–E328.

O'Malley, P., Weir, L., & Clifford, S. (1997). Governmentality, Criticism, Politics. *Economy and Society, 26*(4), 501–217.
Panadol® Australia. (2012). *Manage Your Pain*. Retrieved March 22, 2012, from https://www.panadol.com.au/?cid=SEM:Google:Products_&_Brand_Exact:Brand_-_General&gclid=CJS92eS8uq8CFQcipAodJGfKiQ.
Panksepp, J. (2003). Neuroscience. Feeling the Pain of Social Loss. *Science, 302*(5643), 237–239.
Parsons, T. (1951). Illness and the Role of the Physician: A Sociological Perspective. *American Journal of Orthopsychiatry, 21*(3), 452–460.
Passik, S. D., & Kirsh, K. L. (2004). Assessing Aberrant Drug-Taking Behaviors in the Patient with Chronic Pain. *Current Pain and Headache Reports, 8*(4), 289–294.
Passik, S. D., Kirsh, K. L., & Webster, L. (2011). Pseudoaddiction Revisited: A Commentary on Clinical and Historical Considerations. *Pain Management, 1*(3), 239–248.
Petersen, A. (1997). Risk, Governance and the New Public Health. In R. Bunton & A. Petersen (Eds.), *Foucault, Health and Medicine*. London: Routledge.
Petersen, A., & Lupton, D. (1996). *The New Public Health: Health and Self in the Age of Risk*. London: Sage.
Petersen, A., Davis, M., Fraser, S., & Lindsay, J. (2010). Healthy Living and Citizenship: An Overview. *Critical Public Health, 20*(4), 391–400.
Portenoy, R. K., & Foley, K. M. (1986). Chronic Use of Opioid Analgesics in Non-Malignant Pain: Report of 38 Cases. *Pain, 25*(2), 171–186.
Post, R. M. (2002). Do the Epilepsies, Pain Syndromes, and Affective Disorders Share Common Kindling-Like Mechanisms? *Epilepsy Research, 50*(1–2), 203–219.
Prince, M., Patel, V., Saxena, S., Maj, M., Maselko, J., Phillips, M. R., et al. (2007). No Health Without Mental Health. *Lancet, 370*(9590), 859–877.
Reckitt Benckiser (Australia) Pty Limited. (2010). *Nurofen Pain Relief Advice—Expert Info on Migraines, Headaches, Back Pain, Toothache and More—Targeted Pain Relief with Ibuprofen*. Retrieved March 22, 2012, from http://www.nurofen.com.au/pain-relief/videos/video_player.php?filename=Wedding_Stress.flv&title=Nurofen&transcript=na.pdf.
Robson, P. (2009). *Forbidden Drugs*. Oxford: Oxford University Press.
Rose, N. (2003). The Neurochemical Self and Its Anomalies. In R. V. Ericson & A. Doyle (Eds.), *Risk and Morality*. Toronto: University of Toronto Press.
Royal Australasian College of Physicians. (2009). *Prescription Opioid Policy: Improving Management of Chronic Non-Malignant Pain and Prevention of*

Problems Associated with Prescription Opioid Use. Sydney: Royal Australasian College of Physicians.
Salecl, R. (2004). *On Anxiety*. London: Routledge.
Scarry, E. (1985). *The Body in Pain: The Making and Unmaking of the World*. New York: Oxford University Press.
Searight, H. R., & McLaren, A. L. (1998). Attention-Deficit Hyperactivity Disorder: The Medicalization of Misbehavior. *Journal of Clinical Psychology in Medical Settings, 5*(4), 467–495.
Selye, H. (1950). The Physiology and Pathology of Exposure to Stress: A Treatise Based on the Concepts of the General-Adaptation-Syndrome and the Diseases of Adaptation. *Journal of the American Medical Association, 144*(16), 1414.
Selye, H. (1977). *The Stress of My Life: A Scientist's Memoirs*. Toronto: McClelland and Stewart Toronto.
Shorter, E., & Marshall, J. C. (1997). A History of Psychiatry. *Nature, 386*(6623), 346–346.
Speaker, S. L. (1997). From "Happiness Pills" to "National Nightmare": Changing Cultural Assessment of Minor Tranquilizers in America, 1955–1980. *Journal of the History of Medicine and Allied Sciences, 52*(3), 338–376.
Sporer, K. A., & Kral, A. H. (2007). Prescription Naloxone: A Novel Approach to Heroin Overdose Prevention. *Annals of Emergency Medicine, 49*(2), 172–177.
State Government of Victoria. (2013). *Wellbeing*. Retrieved October 4, 2013, from www.betterhealth.vic.gov.au/bhcv2/bhcarticles.nsf/pages/wellbeing?open.
Stoelting, R. K., & Hillier, S. C. (2012). *Pharmacology and Physiology in Anesthetic Practice*. Philadelphia: Wolters Kluwer Health.
Strong, P. M. (1979). *The Ceremonial Order of the Clinic: Parents, Doctors, and Medical Bureaucracies*. London: Routledge.
Teesson, M., Mitchell, P. B., Deady, M., Memedovic, S., Slade, T., & Baillie, A. (2011). Affective and Anxiety Disorders and Their Relationship with Chronic Physical Conditions in Australia: Findings of the 2007 National Survey of Mental Health and Wellbeing. *Australian and New Zealand Journal of Psychiatry, 45*(11), 939–946.
Teghtsoonian, K. (2009). Depression and Mental Health in Neoliberal Times: A Critical Analysis of Policy and Discourse. *Social Science and Medicine, 69*(1), 28–35.
Tracey, I., & Bushnell, M. C. (2009). How Neuroimaging Studies Have Challenged Us to Rethink: Is Chronic Pain a Disease? *Journal of Pain, 10*(11), 1113–1120.

Turner, B. S. (1984). *The Body and Society: Explorations in Social Theory*. Oxford: Blackwell.

Van de Werf, F., Ardissino, D., Betriu, A., Cokkinos, D. V., Falk, E., Fox, K. A. A., et al. (2003). Management of Acute Myocardial Infarction in Patients Presenting with ST-Segment Elevation. *European Heart Journal, 24*(1), 28–66.

visit4ads. (2012). *Pain Relief with Body Respect Advert, Ad—Panadol Range—Video Clip*. From http://www.visit4ads.com/advert/Pain-Relief-with-Body-Respect-Panadol-Range/91500.

Vrecko, S. (2010). Birth of a Brain Disease: Science, the State and Addiction Neuropolitics. *History of the Human Sciences, 23*(4), 52–67.

Wager, T. D., Atlas, L. Y., Lindquist, M. A., Roy, M., Woo, C.-W., & Kross, E. (2013). An fMRI-Based Neurologic Signature of Physical Pain. *New England Journal of Medicine, 368*(15), 1388–1397.

Williams, S. J., Gabe, J., & Davis, P. (2009). *Pharmaceuticals and Society: Critical Discourses and Debates*. London: Wiley.

Wolf, E. S. (2002). *Treating the Self: Elements of Clinical Self Psychology*. New York: Guilford Press.

World Health Organization. (2014). *WHO Definition of Health*. Retrieved September 10, 2014, from http://www.who.int/about/definition/en/print.html.

Part II

The Way People Experience Non-Medical Use

5

Chilling Out: Recreational and Painkiller Use Among Young People

In a world where social unease and emotional distress are considered to be painful, the use of painkillers has become an ideal response. The desire to escape or manage one's pain thus takes on a new meaning, one that involves the pursuit of pleasure as reprieve from all that ales you in modern life. In alcohol and other drugs literature, the term 'chilling out' often acts as an explanatory tool for the reason why young people engage in recreational drug consumption. The release provided by an inebriated or altered state of mind is a popular way to break from the grind of everyday life. While this has been the case for some time in Western or developed nations, it is important to note significant demographic changes in the consumption of drugs since the countercultural movements of the 1960s.

During the baby boom era, young people in the developed world took to recreational substances in greater numbers (Blackman 1996). Since then, social researchers have focused significant attention on the connection between youth and drug use (Hunt et al. 2010). Contributions from cultural studies (Sulkunen 2002) and subdisciplines such as the sociology of youth (Shildrick 2002) have explored the appeal of recreational drugs for young people to 'relax' via 'escape'—or

G. C. Dertadian, *A Fine Line*,
https://doi.org/10.1007/978-981-13-1975-4_5

'chill out'. In youth culture, the language of 'chilling out' has also emerged as an important way to characterize the process of managing the 'high' of pleasure and the 'low' of pain. The notion of 'chilling out' is embedded in a range of drug-taking practices and youth drug cultures (Blackman 2004), whether it be venues arranging dedicated spaces to 'chill out' (Bellis et al. 2002), users arranging time to 'chill out' while high (Kelly 2007) or engaging in co-use of licit and illicit drugs to 'chill out' your high (Akram and Galt 2009).

While the current study did not focus on young people, recruitment methods did yield a relatively young sample, majority of whom were under the age of 35. This chapter focuses specifically on the experiences of young people because of similarities in the way this group discuss non-medical consumption. The young people in this study spoke about painkillers as being used for recreation or as part of established practices of recreational illicit drug use. For the young people who participated in this study, 'chilling out' was a key reason for their use of recreational and other drugs. This chapter explores the way young people incorporate painkillers into forms of recreational drug use. For some participants this means using painkillers instead of illicit drugs, while for others painkillers are used in various combinations with other drugs.

The chapter starts by addressing the literature on the normalization of illicit drug use, and the way painkillers have come to form part of a similar process for many of the young people who participated in this study. The remainder of the chapter discusses interview data, begging with an assessment of the use of painkillers for 'a numb feeling', in order to avoid general discomfort and emotional worry. The use of pain medications as an intoxicant, or to 'get off your face' is also explored. The chapter then moves to discuss painkiller use when 'coming down' from and managing the 'scary' effects of illicit drug use, finishing with an analysis of the instrumental use of pain medications described by participants.

The Normalization of Drug Use

This chapter provides an empirical discussion about a group of young people (aged 18–30) who use drugs for recreation, and the different roles that painkillers play in this process. The non-medical consumption described includes the use of over-the-counter as well as prescription medications. Some of the data derive from interviews with people over the age of 30, but for whom experiences of painkiller and other drug use occurred largely while aged between 18 and 30. The participants discussed in this chapter represent a set of young people who are familiar with recreational and other forms of drug use. The participants were well educated, all having completed high school. Four hold an undergraduate university degree, and one is enrolled in postgraduate study. They demonstrate an awareness of the properties of the drugs they consume and the effects this might have on their body. For some, this was acquired through formal education (one participant was a chemistry graduate for instance), and for others this knowledge was acquired through social osmosis or personal experience.

Another key observation of this group is that they were experienced drug users. They were all highly familiar with recreational drugs and were either regular consumers or occupied a circle of friends that regularly use 'party drugs' such as MDMA and some psychedelics. For many of those interviewed, painkillers were the drug of choice to provide intoxication, whereas for others painkillers simply mediated the 'high' of other forms of recreational drug use, or managed the health consequences of drug use generally. A significant element of the way participants speak about recreational drug use involves the co-use of illicit drugs and pain medications: what is sometimes referred to as poly-drug use. Given how familiar the sample for this chapter is with recreational consumption, it is useful to canvas research and scholarship about the normalization of drug use to help contextualize aspects of the recreational and analgesic drug consumption of the young people included here.

Research about the normalization of drug use is informed by traditions of critical drugs scholarship. In the early 1960s and 1970s contributions from the sociology of deviance and subcultural theory explored conceptualizations of drug use as 'normal'. Becker (1963) and Young (1971) both rejected then conventional understandings of the 'drug user' as morally and socially 'deviant', preferring instead to produce comparisons between illicit drug use and aspects of 'normal' consumption in society (Measham and Shiner 2009). The continued resonance of the normalization thesis in contemporary research can largely be attributed to convincing empirical evidence that indicates that the proportion of young people who use or come in contact with illicit drugs increased during (and since) the 1960s (Redonnet et al. 2012; Shildrick 2002).

The work of British researcher Howard Parker has been particularly influential in developing current debates about the normalization of illicit drug use among young people. Parker developed a thesis about the changing role of recreational drug use in British youth culture since the 1960s. As part of this thesis, Parker argues that drug use is no longer embedded in rebellious subcultures and that it now forms a 'normal' part of young culture and practice (1998). In a longitudinal study with 465 young adults (aged 18–29), Parker and colleagues accessed: "availability/access; drug trying rates; usage rates; accommodating attitudes to 'sensible' recreational drug use especially by nonusers; and degree of cultural accommodation of illegal drug use" (1998: 941). The research showed that, among other factors, high levels of availability and accessibility of illicit drugs indicate a 'minor normalization' of recreational drug use.

Using Parker's work, Duff has argued for similar trends among Australian youth. However, Duff provides a more conceptual account of normalization, arguing that:

> ...just as young people today grow up painfully aware of the risks and uncertainties of modern life, just as they are taught to exercise judgement and individual responsibility in order to prosper in the new economy, today young people feel capable enough to make their own choices about drugs. (2003: 443)

Duff's argument is grounded in the need to understand the 'meaning and culture' of youth drug use, which, as described above, is thought to be connected to individualized modes of consumption.

A growing set of qualitative data suggests that people who use drugs do exercise a shrewd negotiation of the drug's biological effects, its social character and financial cost (Brain 2000). Many of the participants in this study indicate a similar negotiation of the pharmacology, societal and economic factors related to painkiller consumption and recreational drug use. The impact of, for instance, neoliberal discourse on normalized drug-taking practice is worth elaborating on here. As we shall see throughout the chapter, for many of the participants in this study painkillers are consumed because their status as 'medication' allows for personalized recreation in a broader range of contexts than illicit products would allow.

A Numb Feeling

One of the key motivations for using painkillers non-medically among the young people who took part in this study was for the 'numb feeling' they provide. Participants spoke about the use of painkillers to manage forms of physical and emotional discomfort that was 'numbed' through the effects of the drug. This involved the use of painkillers for mild physical discomfort that did not equate to acute pain, or the use of higher dose or prescription medication that exceeded the relief required for the level of discomfort being experienced. This section will focus in particular on two young men named 'Sean' and 'Collin' who play on the same local inner-city rugby league team together.

Sean is a quick-witted 26-year-old who lives in an inner-city suburb of Sydney. When describing the reasons why he used pain medications, Sean says that they make him feel "*numb in all the right ways*". He described a range of contexts in which he uses painkillers to achieve this numb feeling, some of which include after playing rugby league, when socializing, as well as after a breakup with his girlfriend. The 'rough' atmosphere that constitutes the physicality of the game of rugby league is one example of the kind of reason why Sean might use an over-the-counter medication like Panadol®: "*I always have them after football games*". Sean explained that, while physical discomfort after rugby games did not always warrant the use of pain medication, he would non-the-less use them to be more comfortable as he goes out to socialize after a game: "*And you're all so tough and sore and you wanna go out drinking afterwards*".

Sean also spoke about the use of painkillers for forms of physical discomfort unrelated to sport. He talked about occupying a state of general discomfort:

> Well it's the type of little aches and pains you don't realise you're carrying with you. Like you might have a stiff shoulder. I got a sore back… But just those little cricks that your body has.

When Sean feels these kinds of everyday discomforts, he often takes Panadol® as well as other prescription medication when available:

> It just kind of takes them away, and as a result you just relax as well. Where you might be holding yourself in a certain way, keep[ing] your shoulders straight, you can just kind of sink into it.

This physical numb also provided an emotional relief for Sean, who goes on to say that after taking a painkiller "*you're just like 'ah it's all ok now'*".

The use of painkillers is not, however, Sean's only response to general discomfort. Sean explains that he tended only to use painkillers when they were available or when friends are taking them: "*Most of the time it's—'social' is the wrong word. I see someone else taking something and I'm like 'actually yeah I could probably go for some of that'*". He goes on to provide an example from two years earlier, in which he was returning from a trip away with his then girlfriend:

> We'd just been on a really long drive. It was about eight hours. And we got out of the car and she was complaining about a sore neck from driving and sitting.

Sean recalls that, after his girlfriend decided to take a painkiller:

> I just said "actually, now you mention it I've got a sore back too". Why not. Like I didn't really need one. And we only had Panadeine Forte®, and we said, yeah we'll have that, and if there's a little bit of a buzz to it why not. I think we had a glass of wine as well. We got very relaxed.

Sean presents a blurry line between painkiller use to alleviate discomfort and to experience pleasurable relaxation. Mention of the 'buzz' of the painkiller and its use in combination with alcohol both imply a recreational component to relief from physical discomfort.

One final example of Sean's use for a 'numb feeling' came after he broke up with his long-term girlfriend. Sean used painkillers and other pharmaceuticals to help numb himself from some of the emotional difficulty of the loss:

> I just broke up with my long term partner and I just couldn't sleep. It's like a combination of guilt and sadness. And [the painkiller] wouldn't really affect the sadness that much, but it would help me alleviate the guilt and go to sleep. So I'd just take a temazepam or a Nurofen® when you wake up at 2 in the morning.

For Sean, painkillers did not alleviate the emotion itself, but they did provide a physical sensation that allowed him to cope better with the emotional circumstances. Feeling 'numb' is described as particularly helpful when trying to get back to sleep or get on with the day: '*if the morning was particularly grim, you just take it, just [to] help the day*'. For Sean the 'numb' of the painkiller helped him to cope with what he regarded to be the physical manifestations of his emotions:

> There's definitely a physical component [to strong emotions]. It's just a constant dull pain… The expression heavy heart also comes from that same experience. Because you feel like you're carrying a heavy necklace inside or something. And it's weighing you down.

Sean goes on to say that without the painkiller "*you're still aware of all of the crap*", but when you take a painkiller "*your psyche has a nice warm blanket around it*".

Collin is an easygoing 25-year-old who also spoke about the use of painkillers to deal with a breakup. While backpacking across South East Asia, his girlfriend broke off their relationship via a private message service on the social networking website Facebook:

> It was after a break-up with a girl I had been seeing for two years. Overseas at the time, and so she broke up with me while I was overseas via email, actually via Facebook. It was pretty heart-wrenching, and there was no sense of closure about it.

The lack of closure played on Collin's mind for much of the trip, not being able to properly respond until he returned home:

> So I was left wondering about it for a while. So every morning I'd wake up and there was that couple of seconds before you wake up and you're just normal. Then you remember. And you're instantly upset again.

During the trip, Collin found himself regularly taking benzodiazepines and over-the-counter pain medication: "*I guess maybe subconsciously there was a part of me saying take it because it will make you not upset anymore... You know [a little voice] says take a pill, drink, have some weed*". He described the physical numb provided by the painkiller as particularly useful for avoiding thinking about the breakup before sleep. Collin explained that, on this trip he used painkillers "*as a sedative to get to sleep, 'cause you are kind of kept awake by thinking about it too much*".

The use of painkillers to manage physical/emotional discomfort is a recurring theme among participants. Indeed, most of the young people who participated discussed some element of the alleviation of intertwined physical and emotional unrest; one example of a complex relationship between pain relief and pleasure exhibited by participants. Discussion about a 'numb feeling' was the most explicit reference to forms of drug use that attempt to relieve discomfort *in the body*. Here, 'chilling out' emerges as a form of relaxation that seeks to escape a combination of physical, social and emotional discomfort. For participants who placed a more explicit focus on pleasure, the notion of 'escape' from life circumstances became a significant point of discussion. Use of painkillers for the express purpose of intoxication (or to 'get off your face') forms the focus of the next section.

Getting off Your Face

'Heidi' is a 33-year-old married mother of two boys under the age of 10, who lives in the Western Suburbs of Sydney. Most of Heidi's recreational use of painkillers occurred alongside previous injuries or medical conditions for which she was prescribed strong analgesics. Heidi explains that the recommended dose provided by her prescribing physician was often unsatisfactory to cover her pain, and so she began to exceed the dose:

> [about five years ago] I'd just been in hospital with food poisoning. While I was in emergency they'd given me two Panadeine Fortes®. While it didn't really help, when I was discharged from the hospital they gave me a prescription for another packet of 50 Panadeine Fortes®. So when I got home and I was still having pain I took two, and it wasn't doing much so I took another two and felt that I was a little bit high.

Panadeine Fortes® is a high-dose paracetamol and codeine combination that requires a prescription. Soon Heidi recognized that she enjoyed the pleasurable 'high' she received when using analgesic medications over the prescribed dose and began doing this when the medications became available:

> *Heidi*: I've got a lot problems with my wisdom teeth. I was given Tramadol® for that. So I took the prescribed dose, what I was meant to have, and I thought it was fun so I took more.
> *Researcher*: And why did you take more?
> *Heidi*: Because I wanted to get off my face. High. Because it's fun.

She goes on to explain that this was often a result of boredom. When she was unwell or in pain her partner or parents would take care of her children, which left her with less to do:

> While I was having some pain at the time, I took more than I should have. I just thought I'm taking one for my teeth and I thought 'well I might as well have a few more just to have fun'. Just something to do.

Heidi has also used other drugs recreationally for similar reasons: "*I've always like[d] getting drunk or high or something. I guess it's probably just an escape for a few hours. Just to feel physically and mentally different. It's just a good little break*". Prescription analgesics are described as a way of providing a unique kind of intoxication for Heidi, one different from what she might normally experience: "*I usually drink a lot, [but] I don't smoke dope anymore. [I used Tramadol® because] I just felt like feeling different. Different to usual*". Painkillers are also described as different in social terms:

> It's more of a personal thing. If I was to smoke dope I would do that in front of people and share it, but when I take painkillers it's just a personal thing for me… You can happily go to the bar and buy everyone a drink, but you can't pull out a packet of pills and give everyone a pill. It's a lot different.

She goes on to say that, when using painkillers recreationally, "*I wouldn't be sharing it with anyone. I'd rather just keep that little high to myself. And in myself. I just don't see it as a sharing, social type thing to do*".

Heidi did, however, clarify that "*it depends on who I was with*", explaining that she had used painkillers recreationally with a friend who has "*really bad endometriosis*" (a condition which affects the tissue surrounding the lining of the womb). She recalled that "*I was at this friend's house, we we're drinking beers. She had a bunch of Panadeine Extra®. We crushed up the pills and I showed her how to extract the codeine and we both had that*". Having learnt how to filter codeine out of pharmaceutical products in her teens, Heidi explains the process:

> You just crush up the pills then mix it all together in water. And then filter it through a stocking or a tea-towel or something like that, and everything that goes through to the bottom is codeine and the water and the paracetamol stays on top.

For Heidi, painkillers provided a different kind of 'high', one that broke from the norm and was thus desirable as a form of 'escape'. Her use of painkillers in this way is, however, largely limited to when they have been made available through a legitimate prescription or when a friend decides to share.

Another participant named 'Samantha' also used painkillers for intoxication. Samantha is a 23-year-old Australian with English heritage, who lives in a well-to-do suburb on Sydney's north shore. At the time of interview, she had recently entered a postgraduate program at the university where she completed undergraduate study. Samantha was first introduced to morphine after a surgical procedure she underwent several years earlier:

> I had a PCA (patient-controlled analgesia) monitor after the operation for 12 hours. And so I was hitting it really hard. It was safe because it was in a controlled environment 'cause I was in the hospital. And that kind of gave me a taste for it.

Once she was released from the hospital Samantha explained that she kept "*chasing the feeling*" she had while using morphine.

After leaving hospital, Samantha started to use Panadeine Forte® to help cope with an eating disorder she developed around the same time: "*I would binge and then purge. If I couldn't make myself vomit then I'd want to have pain medication to knock myself out so that I could sleep for ages*". Not only did the prescription analgesic provide a euphoric feeling, it also acted as a sedative that Samantha used to manage the effects of binge eating. She explained that going to sleep right after eating was desirable because "*when I woke up it would feel like my body had digested it*".

Samantha also explained that the 'high' she experienced on Panadeine Forte® was particularly good, especially when compared to forms of illicit intoxication. Previous experiences with illicit drugs have left the impression that they can be, what she described as a ‘dirt high’, and she considered pharmaceutical opiates to be ‘clean’ by comparison. Previous experiences with ecstasy and methamphetamine have left a negative impression of illicit drugs: “*You can have pills or meth, it’s really dirty. And you can kind of feel that it’s really dirty. I swear that before when I used to take ridiculous amounts of pills I felt my brain shaking my skull*”. By comparison, pharmaceutical opiates are described as ideally consistent:

> But when you have something that is opiate based, especially if it’s prescription medication you know that it’s clean… I’ve had pretty much every drug you can have and it’s the ultimate drug that you can have. It’s just complete bliss. It’s amazing. It’s just one constant feeling the whole time. And then it just wears off.

Both the sedative and euphoric qualities of the Panadeine Forte® kept Samantha using the medication for several months after leaving the hospital.

After approximately four months of this kind of sedative/recreational use, Samantha discovered a stock of Panadeine Forte® that her mother had gathered from left over family prescriptions: “*I just found out where it was and there was just this massive stock there. And so for about a month I just ate my way through all of it*”. Her use of the medication escalated, ultimately culminating in a frightening overdose experience in which she also used the prescription medication Seroquel®, which had been prescribed to her as part of her postoperative treatment:

> In January of this year I had 300 milligrams probably at 8 pm, then wasn’t feeling it. Then had another 300 milligrams. You normally only have to wait half an hour to get the effect, but I wasn’t getting the effect, so I had another 300 milligrams. So I had three times my dose, I had pretty much a thousand milligrams of Seroquel®. The immediate release, not the standard release. And then I felt myself OD’ing. ‘Cause I’ve OD’ed before, so I knew how it felt. And I went into my mum. I said “I’ve just overdosed”. My mum gave me heaps of salt water, trying to make me vomit.

After a close call overdose experience, Samantha decided she needed to stop using them: "*mum found out that I'd been going through this stash. And there wasn't any more left and she was really really upset. And then I kind of had to stop 'cause I knew that I would die because of my liver*".

On reflecting about her time using painkillers, Samantha is critical of dominant medical and popular discourses that implicate emotional instability as a reason for recreational use. She explains:

> *Samantha*: Well I suppose they [doctors] would say that you use because you had emotional issues.
> *Researcher*: They might say that, but does that connect for you?
> *Samantha*: They might say that. But honestly… I just use because I like the feeling and that is a really selfish thing to do. I don't think it's any deeper than that… I'm just seeking that feeling.

Samantha also dismisses the role her eating disorder, and associated emotions, may have played in her use of Panadeine Forte®:

> honestly I would love to be able to say "I use because I had childhood abuse" or "shitty self-esteem [about my body]". Which is what doctors tell me, but I honestly think that my use is just really really superficial.

In reflecting about why Samantha used painkillers for intoxication, she says that it is "*just something to do*".

Escaping from boredom is a key feature of alcohol and other drug (Boys et al. 2001) and sociological (Brake 2013) literature. Much of this literature, however, focuses on populations of young men. The 'deviant' status of illicit drug use is thought to make the practice more appealing to groups of young men who enjoy taking risks (Collison 1996). Young men who use drugs are often described in the literature as performing a masculine bravado that revels in risk taking. The examples of Heidi and Samantha, however, demonstrate that this kind of drug use is not simply a masculine pursuit. The gendered elements of Heidi and Samantha's experience are worth noting. Heidi's life is usually bound up in child rearing and its associated responsibilities. However, when she becomes ill and care for the children falls to her partner, Heidi is left with "*nothing to do*": this is when she uses painkillers and other drugs. Samantha's use of painkillers to manage elements of an eating disorder also involves a gendered component. Here, body image and boredom collide as Samantha uses painkillers to "*knock myself out*" after binge eating because "*it makes me feel better*". The next sections explore the way participants use painkillers to help slow the effects of or come down from illicit drugs.

Changing It Up

So far this chapter has explored the use of pain medications as an intoxicant. It has described how a group of young people use painkillers for some form of intoxication, and often within a repertoire of other drugs. This section and the one that follows focus specifically on participants who use illicit drugs to 'get high', but also take painkillers to 'mellow' or reduce intoxication. This includes the use of prescription painkillers to produce a 'different' high, as well as use to help 'come down' from illicit drugs—both of which are practices that a participant named 'Tom' engaged in.

Tom is a 30-year-old backpacker who has been traveling across Australia for the past 5 years. He spoke about taking high-dose analgesics that require a prescription in Australia at various stages during periods (several days) of cocaine and MDMA consumption. Tom crushes up prescription painkillers and combines them with cocaine for a "*gentler*" high. This is mainly done after a long stretch of cocaine use where "*I wanted to keep it going, but I know I could probably do with a bit of a more mellow buzz*". In order to avoid reduced excitement, or risk "*peaking too early*", Tom intervenes by combining painkillers with cocaine to "*change it up*".

Tom also spoke about the use of painkillers toward the end of a "*big night*" on MDMA. He explains that oral painkiller use would help "*wind down the party*" and allow him to go to sleep:

> you'd take them just after a night, if you wanted to go to sleep. Or maybe you've taken so much that you need to chill-out or something

> afterwards, so you stop taking the cocaine or 'e' and then you take maybe a Diazepam® or a Tramadol® just to chill out and relax.

Use of prescription medication to "*chill out and relax*" toward the end of the night also extended to the morning after in some instances:

> I remember one particular time… everyone went out that night and the next morning the sun was coming up and the party was still going. We decided to take the party outside and we were still drinking out there. And a friend, she was a nurse in an old folks home, so she had access to Valium® and Oxy and stuff. And we had a few of them going round and I can remember just lying in the grass just watching a couple of swallows flying about. Just easing out of the party mode.

Descriptions of painkiller use to mellow or wind down illicit intoxication were also discussed by other young people interviewed for this study.

Collin, who was introduced earlier, also used painkillers to manage "*freak outs*" (mild psychosis) when using "*magic mushrooms*" (psilocybin mushrooms). Where Tom was getting bored of the high, Collin describes feeling anxious because of the effects of the drug and thus used painkillers to make sure he could enjoy the experience. Collin recalls using hallucinogenic mushrooms on a road trip with friends to a national park:

> It came on very strongly. Having had the experience before, I knew that it was going to be ok, but you can't get rid of the anxiety that comes with it - just because it's a natural chemical response to hallucinogens.

Having had some medication left over from his trip to South East Asia, Collin brought an assortment of analgesics and anxiolytics (antianxiety agents) with him just in case. Collin explained:

> And so the meds, that we'd actually bought in Laos, we took with us that day as a backup, if we felt anxious. And I did, so I took it, and it

> transformed me. Because I wasn't having much fun 'cause I was a bit too freaked out. And then ten minutes later I was just down with it.

This was something Collin recommended for use with all kinds of hallucinogens, remarking "*it works well in conjunction with acid if you get anxiety with it at all. It takes the scariness out of the experience*". Collin recalled previous experiences where he did not have access to any medication to regulate his use of hallucinogens and emphasized his inability to enjoy those experiences. Bringing the "*meds*" leftover from Laos meant "*it just makes the whole experiences more pleasant*".

Tom and Collin used painkillers as a way to improve their experiences on illicit drugs. Painkillers provided a pharmacological complement to the drugs they consumed that "*changes up the high*" (Tom). These young men describe painkillers as "*safe*" (Collin) and "*trustworthy*" (Tom) and thus as ideal to help alter or adjust their experience when using recreational drugs. The idea that painkillers are relatively benign and largely reliable is a sentiment echoed by many of the participants discussed thus far and also extends to the way participants spoke about the use of painkillers toward the end of the night.

Coming Down

This section explores the use of painkillers when trying to come down off recreational drugs. It discusses the experiences of two young women named 'Bianca' and 'Jane', both of whom use psychoactive drugs intermittently on weekends. Bianca is a 27-year-old participant who spoke about using painkillers after a "*big night*" when using illicit drugs. She is an administrative officer at a large company and has suffered from a painful condition called Familial Mediterranean Fever since her mid-teens. The condition flares up unexpectedly and is often difficult to predict. This has meant that Bianca has been prescribed a wide range of pain medications and is very familiar with the effects these drugs have on her body. While her use of prescription painkillers related mostly to this condition, she did also speak about the use of painkillers in the context of recreational drug use.

Bianca spoke in particular about taking painkillers such as Nurofen® when trying to "*come down*" while using "*ecstasy*". While Bianca's preference was to use sleeping pills, when none are available she takes leftover painkillers to try and get some sleep after a big night out: "*If I had no sleepers [sleeping pills] left and I needed to like calm myself down or relax to sleep. Even just Nurofen® or I get Tramadol®*". Much of the time her use of amphetamines occurred in conjunction with a night out in clubs and bars in night-time entertainment districts in Sydney. Bianca recalls that she uses painkillers "*after taking illicit drugs or something, when we're out dancing and whatever all night, 'cause it's got the calming effect so it helps to put you to sleep*". The analgesic effect is described as useful in a kind of renormalization of a bodily state that will allow sleep: "*[painkillers] just have a kind of analgesic effect on my body. So it does help when you're coming down*". Though Bianca recognized that painkillers are not the ideal mechanism to reverse the effects of amphetamines and that she was not taking them under ideal circumstances, they did provide "*the closest thing*" to a solution for her.

A participant named Jane also spoke about the use of painkillers in a similar. Jane is a soft-spoken 26-year-old who lives in the Eastern Suburbs of Sydney. She described a confident knowledge of how painkillers work and what they can be used for:

> I've definitely given pain medication to friends when they were in pain… and told them about like how pain medication works. Like a lot of people are really ignorant about different things.

She would also often educate friends on the "*active property in different stuff*" informing them that "*they can't combine these things, but that they can combine these things*". An example of Jane sharing her acquired wisdom with a friend is below:

> Like recently a friend of mine had really bad tooth pain, she had exposed nerves, and didn't have the money to go to the dentist immediately… So

> I was helping [her] juggle… Nurofen® [and] Panadeine [Forte]®. I was like 'You have to eat when you have Nurofen®!' She didn't even know that.

This confident knowledge of the effects of analgesic medications informed the way Jane used them with illicit drugs. Jane explains:

> I've mainly used codeine combined with paracetamol or Nurofen®, over-the-counter, in order to get to sleep. When I've had a big night or - yeah, just to get to sleep, or just calm myself down… Mainly it would be using amphetamines, so it would be dexamphetamines or MDMA. Anything that was in my system that was keeping me awake. So if I wanted to counter that.

She goes on to describe one particular time she used painkillers after taking MDMA a few months earlier:

> So I think I remember my ex-partner and I were at his house and we'd had, like sort of a psychedelic. And after quite a few hours of being high we wanted to go to sleep. Some of the effects of what we'd taken weren't very nice… we were in a safe place, with each other, but we were ready to go to sleep and finish the night.

Jane was, however, clear that "*I don't use them all the time*", but prefers having them with her "*in case something goes wrong*". She explains that "*I can remember more like just being prepared. It's like part of my medical kit if anything goes wrong, that's there if I need it, or if anyone I know needs it*".

Jane recalls that her use of painkillers in combination with recreational drugs is one way she manages the illicit context of her consumption. This is informed by a reluctance to rely on the medical profession when engaging in illicit drug use: "*I don't want to have to go to an emergency ward or whatever and tell them what I've taken. And it's never really that bad, so I don't really need to anyway*". To avoid the assumed stigma of an encounter with a medical practitioner, Jane takes a "*just in case*" approach by bringing painkillers along when she knows she (or her friends) will be taking illicit drugs.

Instrumental Use

The young people included in this chapter describe a highly instrumental use of pain medications. They engage in purposeful and considered decisions about the use of these medications for intoxication, or to manage intoxication. An evolving set of literature has dealt with the notion that drug use is a normal practice among young people, which includes functional (as opposed to dependent) use for predetermined purposes other than illicit intoxication (Müller and Schumann 2011; Boys et al. 2001). This facilitates conscious decision making about the use of psychoactive substances for a practical purpose, including to stay awake while driving trucks at long distances (Girotto et al. 2013), to lose weight (Gritz and Crane 1991), help concentrate while studying (McAuliffe et al. 1984) as well as for better sex (Bourne et al. 2015; O'Byrne and Holmes 2010). While much of this disparate set of literature focuses on the functional and instrumental use of illicit drugs, less attention has been paid to the use of pharmaceuticals in this way.

Participants in this chapter describe the instrumental use of pain medications to 'chill out' in a range of contexts. Existing within normalized cultures of youth drug use, the type of painkiller consumption described in this chapter suggests an extension of the neoliberal imperative for individualized approaches to drug use. Participants understand the effects of the painkillers they take and make purposeful choices about how to use them for a combination of overlapping reasons.

The practices described by participants that co-use pharmaceutical and illicit drugs indicate a significant overlap between the pursuit of pleasure and safety. Descriptions about the pleasurable aspects of illicit intoxication are tied closely to its perceived safety. For instance, Tom used painkillers concurrently with other illicit drugs to slow the pace of long periods of cocaine use. Collin used analgesics, among other medications, to reduce the anxiety-producing elements of hallucinogens. Bianca's use of sleeping pills and painkillers make sure she can get to sleep after a big night. Jane prepares for possible risks to her and her friends' well-being by making sure that painkillers are available as a precaution. These kinds of practices are produced, at least in part, by the criminalized context of illicit drug use. Participants sought to avoid the moralizing gaze of medical practitioners and the aggressive and punitive approach of police officers; they take up the use of painkillers to compensate for the lack of provision of health and safety usually deemed to be the responsibility of medical and policing services.

For many of the young people discussed here, painkillers are thus also associated with limiting or retreating from conviviality and sociability. In the context of recreational consumption, painkillers are associated with the private rather than the public sphere. The 'privacy' of painkillers—juxtaposed with the sociality of recreational drugs—also involves a politics of care. Painkillers are used instrumentally to numb, come down, 'make safe' and allow sleep. The 'safety' analgesics provide involves an element of soothing or reassurance. The 'soothing' status of painkillers, as drugs used in private or to comfort, means they are an easy complement to normalized practices of recreational consumption to chill out.

Here, neoliberal faith in the creative capacity of the individual seems in full operation. For instance, for Sean and Collin painkillers are a readily available and cost-effective alternative to illicit drugs. Analgesics also provide other benefits such as the alleviation of physical and emotional discomfort, allowing Collin to socialize after a sports game and Sean to continue to enjoy his trip after a difficult breakup. Similarly, Heidi and Samantha use painkillers to 'change up' their lives and intoxication experiences. The ready availability of analgesics makes them appealing for Heidi to reduce boredom when unwell, while for Samantha analgesics were a 'clean' alternative to illicit drugs. Concurrent analgesic and cocaine use allow Tom to manage his 'high' and sustain his recreation. For Bianca and Jane, painkillers provide a way to control illicit intoxication, and to do so without having to face the stigma of visiting a physician. These are examples of personalized consumption developed to avoid the perceived pitfalls of illicit consumption. Within these examples, neoliberalism appears less as imposing discourse and more as an embedded part of normalized practices of drug consumption.

In discussions with young people, illicit and analgesic drugs are also presented as comparable with the consumption of other consumer products. Young people talk about non-medical and recreational drug use in ways that understand painkillers to be a product for consumption in the neoliberal enterprise of free markets. In this context, painkillers become normalized products for free consumption in the pursuit of 'down time'.

Conclusion

Analgesics are an everyday resource that participants can relatively easily incorporate into their drug-taking practice to enhance it, as well as make it safer. The examples presented thus far represent a significant departure from much of the current epidemiological literature about non-medical consumption, which focuses on the intravenous use of pain medications. For the group of participants discussed in this chapter, intravenous use and 'addiction' do not feature as a concern—if mentioned at all, injecting or dependent consumption was only discussed in passing. Instead, recreational and non-medical drug use forms a relatively mundane and unproblematic element of the lives of the majority of the young people who participated in this study.

This chapter has explored the role that painkillers play in experiences of recreational and illicit drug use among a sample of young people. It has discussed the way painkillers are used as intoxicants that provide a 'numb feeling' and allow participants to feel rested, 'get off their face', and manage their recreational state. While these practices largely refer to forms of recreational release to 'chill out', it is also key to note how they are tied to the alleviation of forms of physical and emotional discomfort. Likewise, the use of painkillers to 'come down' from other forms of illicit intoxication involves an important component of managing physical discomfort, such as a racing heart. Such examples of painkiller consumption can be thought of as part of the contextual normalization of drug use among groups of young people. The painkiller is an everyday product that is an easy addition to the repertoire of recreational and poly-drug use of many young people.

Pleasure is also an important part of why and how young people use painkillers. For the young people discussed in this chapter, the consumption of painkillers was often tied to some form of pleasurable inebriation. Collin and Sean describe a pleasurable 'numb', while Heidi and Samantha talk about enjoying 'being out of it'. Yet for others, like Tom, Bianca and Jane painkillers are used to manage pleasurable experiences with illicit drugs. It is key to note that, for many of the young people who participated in this study painkillers are not static objects whose utility is fixed to social contexts and subjective associations. Painkillers serve shifting purposes that change from one context to another.

The examples outlined here also hint at the presence of a range of structures external to drug use itself. Participants manage physical and emotional pain through forms of medication consumption endorsed by aspects of medical discourse, youth culture and commercial advertising. For instance, for participants like Collin and Jane the level of pleasure experienced when using illicit drugs is tied to their ability to feel or be 'safe': painkillers provide both the ability to experience illicit pleasure and to be safe while doing so. Analgesic use for a pleasant 'escape' is also comparable to medical and commercial discourse about the medication of emotional pain. Participants spoke about how pleasurable intoxication can "pick you up a bit" (Heidi), and "make you feel better" (Collin). These are salient examples of the way broadened understandings of pain impact upon contemporary drug-taking practices.

The next chapter will explore the relationship between recreational drug use (both licit and illicit) and periods of productive work. It builds on the conceptual discussion of the normalization of illicit drug use by exploring how forms of drug consumption are encouraged as a reward for 'hard work'. In particular, it discusses empirical examples of how painkillers are used to enhance both productive work and related recreational release.

References

Akram, G., & Galt, M. (2009). A Profile of Harm-Reduction Practices and Co-Use of Illicit and Licit Drugs Amongst Users of Dance Drugs. *Drugs: Education, Prevention and Policy, 6*(2), 215–225.

Becker, H. S. (1963). *Outsiders: Studies in the Sociology of Deviance*. London: Free Press of Glencoe.

Bellis, M. A., Hughes, K., & Lowey, H. (2002). Healthy Nightclubs and Recreational Substance Use: From a Harm Minimisation to a Healthy Settings Approach. *Addictive Behaviors, 27*(6), 1025–1035.

Blackman, S. (2004). *Chilling Out: The Cultural Politics of Substance Consumption, Youth and Drug Policy*. Maidenhead: McGraw-Hill Education.

Blackman, S. J. (1996). Has Drug Culture Become an Inevitable Part of Youth Culture? A Critical Assessment of Drug Education. *Educational Review, 48*(2), 131–142.

Bourne, A., Reid, D., Hickson, F., Torres-Rueda, S., & Weatherburn, P. (2015). Illicit Drug Use in Sexual Settings ('Chemsex') and HIV/STI Transmission Risk Behaviour among Gay Men in South London: Findings from a Qualitative Study. Sexually Transmitted Infections.

Boys, A., Marsden, J., & Strang, J. (2001). Understanding Reasons for Drug Use Amongst Young People: A Functional Perspective. *Health Education Research, 16*(4), 457–469.

Brain, K. (2000). *Youth, Alcohol, and the Emergence of the Post-Modern Alcohol Order.* London: Institute of Alcohol Studies.

Brake, M. (2013). *The Sociology of Youth Culture and Youth Subcultures: Sex and Drugs and Rock 'n' Roll?* New York: Routledge.

Collison, M. (1996). In Search of the High Life: Drugs, Crime, Masculinities and Consumption. *British Journal of Criminology, 36*(3), 428–444.

Duff, C. (2003). Drugs and Youth Cultures: Is Australia Experiencing the 'Normalization' of Adolescent Drug Use? *Journal of Youth Studies, 6*(4), 433–446.

Girotto, E., Mesas, A. E., de Andrade, S. M., & Birolim, M. H. (2013). Psychoactive Substance Use by Truck Drivers: A Systematic Review. *Occupational & Environmental Medicine, 71*, 1–6.

Gritz, E. R., & Crane, L. A. (1991). Use of Diet Pills and Amphetamines to Lose Weight Among Smoking and Nonsmoking High School Seniors. *Healthy Psychology, Health Psychology, 10*(5), 330–335.

Hunt, G., Moloney, M., & Evans, K. (2010). *Youth, Drugs, and Nightlife*. London: Routledge.

Kelly, B. C. (2007). Club Drug Use and Risk Management Among "Bridge and Tunnel" Youth. *Journal of Drug Issues, 37*(2), 425–443.

Measham, F., & Shiner, M. (2009). The Legacy of 'Normalisation': The Role of Classical and Contemporary Criminological Theory in Understanding Young People's Drug Use. *International Journal of Drug Policy, 20*(6), 502–508.

McAuliffe, W. E., Rohman, M., Fishman, P., Friedman, R., Wechsler, H., Soboroff, S. H., et al. (1984). Psychoactive Drug Use by Young and Future Physicians. *Journal of Health and Social Behavior, 25*(1), 34–54.

Müller, C. P., & Schumann, G. (2011). Drugs as Instruments: A New Framework for Non-Addictive Psychoactive Drug Use. *Behavioral and Brain Sciences, 34*(6), 293–310.

O'Byrne, P., & Holmes, D. (2010). Desire, Drug Use and Unsafe Sex: A Qualitative Examination of Gay Men Who Attend Gay Circuit Parties. *Culture, Health & Sexuality, 13*(1), 1–13.

Parker, H. (1998). *Illegal Leisure: The Normalization of Adolescent Recreational Drug Use*. London: Taylor & Francis.

Redonnet, B., Chollet, A., Fombonne, E., Bowes, L., & Melchior, M. (2012). Tobacco, Alcohol, Cannabis and Other Illegal Drug Use among Young Adults: The Socioeconomic Context. *Drug and Alcohol Dependence, 121*(3), 231–239.

Shildrick, T. (2002). Young People, Illicit Drug Use and the Question of Normalization. *Journal of Youth Studies, 5*(1), 35–48.

Sulkunen, P. (2002). Between Culture and Nature: Intoxication in Cultural Studies of Alcohol and Drug Use. *Contemporary Drug Problems, 29*(2), 253–276.

Young, J. (1971). *The Drugtakers: The Social Meaning of Drug Use*. London: MacGibbon and Kee.

6

Work Hard, Play Hard: Cycles of Restrain and Release in Painkiller Use

The significance of working hard in order to achieve financial success has long been a central organizing principle of capitalism. Diligent work and financial security are often accompanied by a sense of purpose and pride in oneself. Of course, with the advent of mobile computing and online enabled technology work has intensified, and as is symptomatic of the fragmentation of late-modern societies, it has become also less secure. The centrality of work in modern life also has implications for leisure and recreation as people seek to escape from the demands of paid employment. The desire to engage in recreational release is linked in important ways to the modern imperative for productivity. The Part One outlined the way medical and commercial interests have turned their attention to the productivity of the modern worker. Where Chapter 5 spoke about the instrumental use of painkillers among a group of young people who engaged in recreational drug use, this chapter focuses on a broader group of participants who use painkillers for productivity and for recreation. It discusses the use of painkillers at work, as well as to manage episodes of 'time out' after work and on weekend break from work.

G. C. Dertadian, *A Fine Line*,
https://doi.org/10.1007/978-981-13-1975-4_6

The chapter draws on interview data from a range of participants in this study, some of whom will be introduced below, and others who have been introduced in the previous chapter. It analyzes participant descriptions of periods of productive work and recreational release as 'reward' for hard work. In doing so, the chapter outlines a framework for understanding the consumption of painkillers to enhance everyday cycles of restraint and release in, what is referred to as a 'work hard, play hard' dynamic.

The chapter begins by articulating a conceptual framework about neoliberalism and modern work. Utilizing this framework, the chapter then explores a series of empirical examples of painkiller consumption related to productive work. This includes the use of painkillers to 'bulldoze through' physical or emotional discomfort, use to 'deal with stress' and to 'manage sleep'. Less traditional forms of work are also explored through the use of pain medication to 'concentrate while studying' and enhance the performance of domestic labor. The chapter then goes on to discuss the use of pain medications as a form of postwork release in social rituals of 'time out'. A conceptual discussion of the social significance of alcohol consumption as a method of recreation is first addressed, before exploring the empirical examples of participants who use painkillers to 'get more drunk' and as a 'hangover cure'.

Neoliberal Work

A significant theme that emerged out of interviews with participants in the study was the use of painkillers to manage their ability to remain productive at work, and while engaging in less conventional forms of labor. The sections that follow will discuss a series of examples of painkiller consumption for the purpose of productivity. Before elaborating on these empirical examples, this section will articulate a conceptual framework that helps to explain the role of self-governance in consumption conducive to productivity.

The role of the neoliberal philosophy in economic and social policy has had important implications on the structures of modern work and paid employment. As outlined in Chapter 1, neoliberal policies have formed part of processes of macroeconomic reform pursued by governments and a transnational business elite over the last thirty years. Social researchers have also noted that neoliberal emphasis on 'flexibility' in industrial relations has often translated into a reduction in the rights of the individual worker (Smith and Morton 2006; Palley 2005). As a result, the working world is increasing made up of casual and short-term contracts. The requirement to work harder and to demonstrate your worth to current and prospective employers, who are under fewer obligations to provide stable working conditions, is now one of the lived realities of neoliberal work.

Fractured and uncertain employment also impacts on the way work is governed and experienced. Short-term and casual contract work has made employment less secure in industrial societies (Barbieri 2009; Bauman 2007). Advances in computing and communication technology have also played a significant role in reshaping experiences of and expectations about work. The enhanced role of the internet and a proliferation of mobile computing devices have increased the speed and expanded the terrain of 'work' (Freeman 2002; Baily and Lawrence 2001). These conditions of employment invariably inform the way work is experienced. Indeed, the demands of modern work are increasingly described as stressful and headache inducing (Harkness et al. 2005), and an entire research literature has developed around the "work stress 'epidemic'" (Gregg 2011; Wainwright and Calnan 2000).

Levels of stress at work, and the bodily responses that accompany stress, have also been presented as impediments to the productivity of the modern worker. Political rhetoric has constantly represented the productivity of the Australian workforce as being in decline "since the record highs of the 1990s" (Parham 2012: vii). Medical and commercial responses to stress-induced-illness or discomfort often foreground biological considerations. Chapter 4 already outlined how medical discourses present (headache) pain as an impediment to self-expression and social participation. It also outlined how consumer discourse borrows from the notion of pain as an obstructing force, positioning the purchase and consumption of over-the-counter analgesics as a remedy to pain's obstruction of self-fulfillment. Many direct-to-consumer advertisements for over-the-counter painkillers involve depictions of office workers who are incapacitated by the pain of a headache. Alongside the relief of physical pain, the consumption of Panadol® or Nurofen® is also presented to be a way to return to the worker the capacity to be productive.

By presenting stress as an individual biological response with a pharmaceutical solution, medical and consumer discourse can obscure the social determinants of work-related-stress. This process borrows from long traditions of medicalization that construct socially undesirable or inconvenient bodily responses as medical symptoms (Conrad and Schneider 1992). However, the increased commercialization of medical discourse introduces a new element to the landscape of medicalization scholarship, with a focus on 'pharmaceuticalization' introduced to aid in the analysis of the entanglement of medical and consumer discourse.

Sociologist Melinda Cooper (2008) has argued that the 'neoliberal turn' during the 1980s coincided with a series of creative transformations and technological advances in the life sciences. Cooper notes that the technological advancements in molecular, cellular and microbiology during the era of neoliberal reform have created an "intense traffic between the biological and the economic spheres" (2008: 4). As a result, medical, biological and economic development over the last thirty years has often involved shared interests, skills and social networks. This has fostered a close relationship between the medical profession and the biotechnology and pharmaceutical industries (Clarke et al. 2003).

Overlap between medical and commercial interests has also informed analysis about the medicalization and pharmaceuticalization of productivity at work. In theorizing the use of medications in contemporary working environments, Keane observes:

> Discourses of productivity and flexibility construct a regulatory ideal of an adaptable, alert, multitasking worker… At the same time the discourses of enterprise and excellence that have flourished in neoliberal economies emphasise the continual improvement of work performance… One consequence of these trends is the problematisation and medicalisation of traits that interfere with optimum performance and efficiency. (Keane 2011: 109)

Keane elaborates on the role of the individual in negotiating these processes of medicalization by borrowing from Rose's notion of 'biological citizenship': a concept which suggests that the individual is made responsible for and becomes responsive to biological considerations (Rose 2009). Keane argues that, as a result of neoliberal influences on working conditions "pharmaceutical self-management [has become] an attribute of the responsible worker" (Keane 2011: 117).

The convergence of medical and consumer discourse in the context of neoliberal working conditions has promoted the desirability of a pharmaceutically induced productivity. The sections that follow will provide a series of empirical examples of painkiller consumption related to productivity and work. The examples outlined in this chapter do not form a direct relationship with biomedical frameworks for medication consumption: instead they borrow from and appropriate contemporary forms of legitimate medical discourse.

Bulldozing Through

The need to stay productive at work in the face of physical illness or in anticipation of illness was a significant point of discussion among participants. Some participants spoke about the preemptive use of painkillers to avoid feeling unwell. 'Tony', a 28-year-old Operations Manager from Perth, spoke about the use of painkillers to remain productive at work in particular detail. Tony is single and takes his job very seriously, doing most of his work from behind a desk in the inner-city office of the company he works for: "*I work 8 hours a day, five days a week, staring at a screen*". His job involves managing a small team of people to meet tight deadlines.

Tony's work was often a cause of headache inducing stress, and painkillers play an important role in making sure he could keep working. The kinds of physical discomfort that result from his work included "*dizziness*" and a "*throbbing forehead*": "*it's like a small dizzy spell or just a throbbing from staring at the screen for too long without taking a break*".

Tony also spoke about the use of painkillers in anticipation of feeling unwell: "*if I'm starting to feel even slightly unwell I'll take a couple [of Panadols®], just to try and sort of bulldoze through*". Tony explained that he commonly used Panadol® to 'bulldoze through':

> There has probably been several occasions… where I've been working, working, working, staring at the screen for say an hour or two at a time and I don't know like - it is just almost like a faint feeling in my head. It wasn't quite tiredness, but it was just like lack of energy almost. But just felt slightly disorientated and I guess the first reaction was to go and grab a couple of Panadols from the staff cupboard.
>
> If I start to feel like a spell coming on the first thing I normally do, without normally doing anything else, is to start going into the kitchen and grabbing a couple of Panadol®. And look normally it works. Just as I said bulldozes through. Whether it is an actual headache or it's something else, the Panadol® just sort of bulldozes through anything really.

For Tony, Panadol® is an entirely innocuous device he uses to get through the day, and the workplace itself provided a legitimizing context for this kind of consumption. The staff cupboard is "*always stocked*" with Panadol® and employees are free to consume its contents with little to no scrutiny from management. Though Tony conceded that a short walk and some fresh air might have the same effect, a pharmaceutical intervention is usually the most convenient option for him to maintain productivity.

A 35-year-old office worker from Sydney named 'Michael' also used painkillers when trying to regulate his productivity. Michael is employed on multiple casual and part-time contracts for companies in different industries. This makes for a busy schedule that often leaves him tired and run down. When explaining a particularly stressful week that had just gone past, Michael recalls:

> It was probably on Sunday. No it was Saturday. I had to do something or meet somebody. I've been to too many work-places this week. Yeah I was just thinking am I going to be able to cope getting up on a Saturday?

Having already had a busy week, Michael was worried about his ability to perform at a meeting on Saturday morning. He contemplated taking a painkiller to help him sleep, but decided against it to avoid "*feeling groggy*" in the morning and "*looking a bit sloppy*" at the meeting. Instead, Michael took some Panadol® the morning of the meeting: "*So I took it before I left and had my coffee and got motivated to work*".

Michael describes himself as "*hyperactive*" and said that is sometimes an impediment to his work. He explained "*I'm one of those people who picks up a lot and sees a lot. I'm very hyperactive as it is*" and that painkillers help to "*shut that hyperactivity down*". Michael goes on to describe how his use of painkillers to dull hyperactivity helped him 'get in the zone' for a period of productive work. He says that he sometimes takes painkillers "*Just to blank out. It blanks out a headache. I just [take] four before work 'cause I just wanted to be in the zone*". Recalling one morning where he had a lot to do, Michael took Nurofen® "*before I left [for work] and had my coffee and knew I would be motivated*".

When using painkillers before work Michael preferred to take Nurofen® because:

> I don't usually dump pain relievers with water, it's usually like straight down the hatch. With Panadol® it was like 'errk.' But those [Nurofen® tablets] were like sugar… they tasted like lollies to me.

His preference for Nurofen® is explained as such: "*I'm highly addicted to sugar. So anything with a bit of sugar in it. [Nurofen®'s] got that sort of a bit sweetish, or better flavour*". Michael did, however, go on to describe some contradictory feelings about his use of Nurofen®. Due in part to a back injury he sustained several years earlier, Michael began using Nurofen® on a regular basis for a period of approximately two years, which he says was "*doing a lot of damage*". Three years prior to interview Michael was diagnosed with reflux after an uncomfortable night he had to visit to the local hospital's emergency ward: "*The stomach was leaking. And that was due to using too much iBuprofen for about a period of two years*". While Michael now uses Nurofen® more judiciously, he will often keep it in mind if he has a busy schedule.

Dealing with Stress

Work-related-stress is also a key motivation for painkiller use among participants. While stress was an important part of the way Tony and Michael use painkillers preemptively, a participant named 'Ray' spoke directly about responding to stress by taking painkillers. Ray is a 45-year-old Australian man, who has done shift work for most of his career. A few years ago Ray left a telecommunications company that he had worked for since he was 30: "*I was there for like 10 and a half years, and I was happy for the first seven. Then I probably left it a bit too long to find something else to do*".

Working with difficult customers, usually over-the-phone, proved an unwelcome source of stress for Ray: "*it was always 'what nasty customer am I going to get today?' So you always think something bad is going to happen*". But it was not just the customer that put Ray on edge at his previous job. He recalls that:

> I work[ed] with people that, if they got a nasty customer, they would just genuinely explode. Thump the desk. Start screaming "fuck this! fuck that!" And then run off half mad and have a cigarette.

When Ray felt intimidated by the situation, he often took painkillers to relax: "*It just made me numbed for a bit, made me more relaxed. So that if they blow up I can just think 'its nothing to do with you. Relax. Don't take it personally'*".

Since leaving his former employer, Ray has taken casual shift work as a security guard. His use of painkillers has been less frequent in this position, though he does still take them when they are available. With reference to his new job, Ray says: "*If I've run out of them [painkillers], I won't buy more until I'm actually feeling sick. But then if I've got like a box of 24 in my bag, that's when I tend to take them for just stress and things like that*". He mainly takes painkillers before work, as a way to prepare for a difficult day:

> It's not just after something particularly bad has happened. It's usually at the start of the shift and I'm just like, "Don't wonna be here. Gonna

> get a coffee. Have Panadol® with the coffee? Yeah". It just makes sure that you're covered for the shift, if it gets too stressful.

When elaborating on this kind of use to deal with stress, Ray also made comparisons to the way he might consume confectionaries:

> It was about 8'oclock, I started at about 7[pm]... Had a coffee, had a cigarette and then I'm like "I think I have Panadol® in the bag". I didn't have a headache or anything like that. It's just 'cause I had it there and I just remember, it's like having a bag of lollies in the bag or something.

When asked to elaborate on the comparison to a "*bag of lollies*", Ray went on to say: "*I didn't need Panadol® if that makes any sense. I just wanted it. Same way you don't need a jelly snake unless you're diabetic or something. You know, you just want it*". Here Ray highlights the way Panadol (and other over-the-counter analgesics) are used as consumer products. This has important links to the way sociologists have described the connection between medical and commercial discourse. Ray's use of painkillers is a requisite example of the way social (and working) conditions produce forms of social anxiety and suffering, for which consumer products are presented as the solution.

Managing Sleep

Similar accounts of preemptive consumption emerged around the use of painkillers to manage sleep to be alert the next day. Lack of sleep has been described as a significant consequence of work-related stress (Chatzitheochari and Arber 2009), and the harmful consequences of disrupted sleeping patterns are a significant component of the stress literature (Åkerstedt et al. 2002; Steptoe 2006). However, benzodiazepines (commonly referred to as 'sleeping pills' or 'tranquilizers'), not analgesics are most commonly prescribed for the regulation of sleep. Two participants in particular describe the use of painkillers to get a good night's sleep when stressed. This section will elaborate on interviews with a woman named 'Mary', as well as return to aspects of Tony's use of painkillers.

Mary is a 39-year-old Vietnamese-Australian woman who arrived in Australia during her late-teens. The last decade has been a difficult time for Mary, who has a very different life now than she did ten years ago:

> It was very bad before, because I went through divorce, I end up in the criminal refuge because of domestic violence. And I studied at University with my little boy, he was really young, just born. He got sick all the time. My second son passed away. A lot of stress happened in the last ten years.

As the mother of a young boy at primary school, negotiating the burdens of single motherhood and the demands of a fast-paced professional environment is important to Mary. Trying to strike the right balance is a stressful task. When describing the physical sensation that accompanies stress, Mary says:

> Very funny pain when you are stressed. You feel pain but you don't know where. Sometimes it's not a headache, it's not a shoulder, it's not a belly-ache. It's just pain, but you don't know where. That's how the stress comes.

When feeling stressed, painkillers are one of the ways Mary makes sure she can manage her schedule.

Mary has worked in various administrative positions for the better part of 10 years and at the time of interview her job always involved a looming deadline. Recalling a particularly busy period a year earlier, Mary said: "*I [knew] that my schedule tomorrow [was] going to have a deadline… and I was like 'oh no, I need to have a good sleep to prepare for tomorrow'. And I thought I should take a painkiller*". Describing the relief that the over-the-counter analgesic Nurofen® provide when she is stressed out and needs to sleep, Mary says:

> Straight after I'm taking the painkiller, 5 minutes or a couple of minutes after that I feel good. I feel comfortable. Because I already prepared for the stress. Even if the stress is not pain yet I feel comfortable, I feel ready for it. When I go to bed, I take a painkiller and think "ah, I can relax now because I'm gonna have a very good sleep".

Her use of painkillers to get a 'good sleep' forms part of a wider story about her need to be productive. Mary anticipated her schedule and decided whether 'good sleep' is required for productive work the next day: "*I still have to take a painkiller before bed, and during the day if I've got a deadline. You know I have to take it to concentrate*".

Tony also spoke about taking painkillers to regulate sleep, saying that he had not always been so focused on his job. Up until only three years ago, Tony had spent a lot more time with his then partner, who remained an elusive figure in the interview, except to say that he did not take their breakup well. Tony reflected that "*it just made me very sad, because she was just gone and I didn't know what do with that*". Tony threw himself into his work but found it difficult to get into a healthy sleeping pattern: "*I was basically not sleeping at night because me and my partner went our separate ways*".

In an attempt to better regulate his sleeping pattern, Tony went to a general practitioner who prescribed sleeping tablets. While they worked at first, it became difficult to sleep comfortably without them: yet he resolved that "*it was fine, now I've stopped using them as much and it's fine*". One of the other techniques Tony adopted to regulate sleep after the breakup was the use of painkillers: "*You know like on nights where I'm feeling particularly stressed or if I need a good night's sleep or if I haven't been sleeping well lately*". Similar to Mary, the ability to sleep well the night before provides Tony with the certainty that he will be able to concentrate the next day.

Concentrating While Studying

Professional or paid employment was not the only kind of work that participants spoke about. Interviewees also spoke about the use of painkillers to be productive while engaging in unpaid or less traditional forms of labor. For a 25-year-old participant name 'Jason', painkillers are used to assist with levels of concentration when studying for University assignments. Jason was born in Colombia and came to Australia to study in 2008. He has had ongoing issues with his Australian visa and has only been able to secure unstable or casual work. His visa and work situation contribute to stress and anxiety that becomes difficult and distracting when assessments are due:

> I was down a little bit because I was stressed. I was stress because I couldn't find a job, I was stressed because I didn't understand the Units I had to do, the assignments. Everything, the [Australian] system is completely different.

In order to inoculate himself from the stress, Jason uses painkillers: "*I always try to keep medicine in my bag. I always have something in my bag just in case*". He takes painkillers such as Panadol® and Nurofen® to avoid feeling physically run down or getting sick: "*when you feel sad and stressed and stuff like that your body also responds to that, so you feel down and feel you are going to get sick*". He described the effects of painkillers as helping to make his body feel relaxed, making him less susceptible to the discomfort of feeling anxious: "*So sometimes when you take something you know at least the body is going to feel better, even though your thoughts are still going to be there*".

During a period of unstable work a few years earlier, Jason had to move from his apartment unexpectedly. After moving into a new apartment, Jason met a roommate who offered him some Panadeine Forte® to cope with his clashing study commitments:

> Yeah she was also living there and she said "ok I take this one when I'm really stressed… when I have too many assignment and when I have too much University stuff". And she gave me one packet. But it finished very quickly.

Panadeine Forte® helped Jason "*concentrate more*" without "*worry[ing] too much about things and getting headaches*". Jason also worried about his English proficiency and how it affected his performance at university. Recalling a particularly busy period later that year Jason says:

> First of all it was a difficult topic, second it was in English and English is not my native language. So sometime – when you know what you want to say... but you don't know —you don't find the words.

Jason was not working at the time either, and this compounded his concern about the demanding workload: "*Yeah and that makes it more stressful, and the teacher was very very demanding. Was very strict with us. So it was like a lot of things, where I felt like in shock*".

Jason's inability to focus on his University work is linked to a range of circumstances, such as stress from uncertain financial, visa and housing arrangements. His use of painkillers ensured that he can maintain concentration in order to get his work done.

Taking Care of the Kids

For many of the women who participated in this study a significant reason for the non-medical use of painkillers related to their ability to manage domestic responsibilities. The need to find ways to be motivated for and physically able to care for small children was an important theme in the interviews. 'Sarah' is one participant who spoke about the use of painkillers related to her ability to take care of her children. As a young mother of 20-month-old twins, one boys and one girl, Sarah had a lot on her plate at the age of 18. She lives in a rural town in NSW, where she has spent most of her life. After leaving High School in Year 11 to raise her children, Sarah worked odd jobs in retail but often finds it difficult to get a babysitter, which means she has had to rely primarily on her partner's income to support the family.

When describing a particularly difficult day at the funeral of a close family member, Sarah explained that she was having a hard time coping with the stress of the loss while having to take care of the children and deal with some financial issues. During a period of commiseration with her family, Sarah's children were "*just being really naughty and they were sick as well*". To top it all off her partner informed her that he had just lost his job: "*so I was really stressed about money and didn't know what we were gonna do*". The situation became overwhelming and Sarah suspected that it was responsible for the nasty headache that soon developed. She recalled taking prescription analgesic Mersyndol® because it was the only medication offered to her by the family member whose home they were visiting at the time.

Sarah recalled that she did not think that the pain warranted a prescription painkiller, but that the extra strength medication did help her deal with the situation: "*it just let me relax and let me think about the problem better*". The use of Mersyndol® made her more patient with her children at a time when they needed her to be patient: "*like they were sick and upset as well, so after the Mersyndol® I was just like more relaxed and could give them more attention you know*". Sarah goes on to reflect, "*like it didn't really fix the situation or the problems but it made me look at things in a different way*". For Sarah, the extra dose of analgesic allowed her the physical and mental utility to be there for her children. As a result, Sarah also started using prescription analgesics to more thoroughly remove the symptoms of a hangover, so that she would feel up to entertaining her young children the morning after a 'big night'. Use of painkillers to manage a hangover will be dealt with in more detail later on in the chapter.

Other participants also described painkiller consumption as a social cue that could provide productive distance from the responsibilities of taking care of the kids and other domestic duties. The need to 'get away' was an important part of the way some women are able to sustain the demands placed on them. 'Jenny' is a 33-year-old mother of three children who injured her back while serving a tour in the armed forces in her early twenties. She is often prescribed morphine and other analgesics related to the injury and has used them regularly over the last fifteen years.

One of the other main reasons Jenny has used painkillers is the migraines she started to experience after she had children:

> About twelve years ago my first thing, a mother having children I had a lot of headaches, I suffered from migraines and I would take at least eight Nurofen® a day through the day so I wouldn't have a migraine.

Sometimes the combination of her injury and the stress of domestic responsibilities would collide in ways that were particularly difficult. She recalled one time when "*my children were sick. I was sick. I was in pain. And I was around my parents who were just not helping at all... and because the stress had escalated so much that my back had gone out*". On occasions such these, morphine became very useful.

Jenny recalled that a few years prior to interview her use of morphine started to become a bit of a crutch. Due to a range of factors that seemed to collide all at once her use became more frequent: "*Ok, a mother of three, a husband that's in the services that's away a lot. I am an ex-army soldier, there was a lot of things. I didn't have a job, I didn't have an identity*". While much of her use of morphine was still related to the injury, she went on to say that other factors also began to play a role:

> Because [when] I was on it, people knew that I was on it for a reason... It made it easier to just lay around and be in pain I guess. I slept a lot with it so when I slept no one bothered me. No one came and wanted me to do anything so it was easy to escape life.

Jenny went on to explain that her pain has since improved. She has been tapered down to a lower-dose pain medication and is using them less than she used to.

'Jessica' is another participant who had a similar experience to Jenny. Jessica is 41 years old and works a demanding administrative job at a local business. She is also the mother of two young boys under the age of 10. Jessica had been prescribed analgesics for several years in relation to a series of "*clumsy accidents*" while "*camping with the family*" and "*taking the kids for a walk*". However, she also took her prescribed medications when she got migraines: "*Well I suffer from chronic migraines, so a lot of the time I use pain medications for that*". Jessica's migraines are often exacerbated by stress related to domestic responsibilities. She recalled how she used Mersyndol Forte® a few years earlier:

> It would probably have been in the school holidays, 'cause I was on holidays at the same time. [My husband] decided he was going to clean out the fridge so I was taking care of the kids... And he'd pulled everything

> out of the fridge and was wiping the shelves down, but he left the fridge door open and it was beeping. And I said "just shut the fridge door before you clean everything out". And he said "oh no its not bothering me". And I went "yeah but it's really bothering me". So I ended up taking some Mersyndol Forte® and taking myself off to the other side of the house again, just to get away and also to calm down.

She explained, "*so I guess I tend to take the pain medications for stress as well as the pain*".

Jessica also reflected on the complexities of her use of painkillers to de-stress. She wondered about whether her use of analgesics had been motivated by more than simply wanting to ameliorate migraine pain. The way the stress of her domestic life impacted on the presence of migraines was a point of contention. The following exchange from the interview details her concern about migraines and medication consumption:

> *Jessica*: I mean it's possible that the headaches or migraines that I was getting were more psychosomatic.
> *Researcher*: Why would you say that the migraine's were psychosomatic?
> *Jessica*: Just maybe because I was feeling really really tense and was almost expecting a migraine to come. I was almost anticipating it and medicating before-hand.

Here Jessica described a kind of preemptive consumption that is comparable to the way other participants discussed thus far have used painkillers to avoid illness or headache pain at work. However, the discourses of productive consumption that frame the narratives of people who take painkillers to avoid headaches at work are less available to Jessica, whose responsibilities are domestic rather than commercial or professional.

Jessica goes on to explain that her painkiller consumption has now evolved from use for migraine pain to use for relaxation: "*So I was taking the painkillers as an excuse to get away. Whereas now I recognise that 'ok so I need to take something to calm me down'*". It is, however, important to note that there are significant overlaps between the forms of use Jessica described. The presence of migraine pain may provide a legitimizing biomedical framework, but the reasons for Jessica's analgesic consumption remained largely consistent. Though the presence of migraine pain may no longer be necessarily to initiate Jessica's use of pain medications, she still took painkillers "*to relax*" and "*to be left alone*" so that she is better able to fulfill the responsibilities of domesticity and motherhood: "*I just can't keep up unless I have at least some time to myself*".

As noted in the conceptual discussion about work and productivity at the outset of this chapter, medical and consumer discourse form part of neoliberal modes of governance that tacitly endorse pharmaceutical self-management. The empirical examples discussed thus far demonstrate how individual consumers adopt and appropriate socially legitimate notions of biomedical impediment to productive work. Participants in the study anticipate forms of physical discomfort and emotional worry likely to interrupt work, study and domestic responsibility, and they pre-empt it through self-medication.

Neoliberal Play

When the working week is done, it is common to recover and unwind with a night out on the town, often with the goal of intoxication. Intoxication allows for a pleasurable release from the constraints of the working world, which, as we saw above, can demand dedicated periods of restraint for productivity. This kind of 'time-out' ritual has become an important part of contemporary understandings of productivity. Neoliberal notions of productive work are closely comparable to social expectations about recreational consumption. The neoliberal subject is expected to engage in recreation that does not interfere with productive goals. While the previous sections have outlined the way painkillers are used to ensure or enhance productivity, the remainder of the chapter will explore the 'time-out' rituals that foster a continuation of cycles of restraint and release.

Forms of pleasurable 'release' are a central part of contemporary debates about the normalization of drug consumption, which were canvassed in the previous chapter. Research suggests that young people develop an enterprising relationship with the drugs they consume, one that takes into consideration its physiological effects, social identity and financial cost (Brain 2000). The normalization of alcohol consumption does, however, involve a set of specific forms of socialization and involves a different kind of political economy of consumption to that of illicit drug use. Illicit drug use can only be understood as normalized within particular social contexts and among a selection of subcultural groups, many of which are defined by their subversive character: rave culture (Duff2003, 2005), the club drug scene (Fazio et al. 2010; Shacham and Cottler 2010), and street or gang culture (Sanders 2012) are key examples. By contrast, in Australia the consumption of alcohol for the explicit purpose of intoxication is viewed as a widely acceptable, and even expected form of social lubrication (Australian Institute of Criminology 2009).

Contemporary research into alcohol is most often concerned with its consumption among young people in the night-time economy. Speaking about the British context Hobbs writes that:

> Alcohol consumption provides both a culturally and legally sanctioned way of altering behaviour, and it is this opportunity to enjoy legitimised 'time out' in the form of hedonistic forms of experiential consumption and identification, that renders the night-time economy so alluring to young people. (Hobbs 2003)

Similar arguments about the Australian context are well established, with research focusing on alcohol-related violence in the night-time economy (Tomsen 2003). Tomsen and colleagues write that the Australian night-time economy is 'focused around 'time out' periods at night and towards or during the weekend, and are centered on entertainment areas and venues' (1990: 4). Night-time entertainment districts in Australia are thus made up of venues like bars and pubs, designed both socially and economically around the consumption of alcohol (Miller et al. 2013).

The regulation of alcohol has been progressively liberalized for several decades. Australia's road to the liberalization of alcohol gained momentum in the second half of the twentieth century (Filmore and Roizen 2000), which began in the response to tightening regulations on analgesics and other drugs. Recent moves toward the liberalization of alcohol regulation, now available for sale by large supermarkets, seem to confirm the at least partly depoliticized status of alcohol. Forming an important part of the operation of the night-time economy, escapism through alcohol intoxication, often in the form of binge drinking, is now thought to often be "the norm rather than the exception among young people" (Harrison et al. 2011: 469).

Today, the consumption of alcohol is regulated in market-based policy structures that competitively encourage maximum purchase and consumption. Though excessive alcohol use certainly attracts stigmatization (Fortney et al. 2004; Room 2005), the drug itself is largely excluded from such stigmatizing discourses. Despite public controversy surrounding alcohol-related violence, alcohol's at least partly legitimized status means it is still presented as safe in moderation. Consumer and public health discourse present alcohol as safe in moderation and thus permissively endorse its consumption as the drug of choice for social rituals of 'time out'. Public health approaches to alcohol often incorporate the notion of the 'responsible drinker'. Aspects of the public health response to alcohol thus rely on neoliberal notions of the rational consumer, who is required to manage appropriate forms of recreation (Harrison et al. 2011; McCreanor et al. 2005).

Alcohol consumption is a state-sanctioned and socially acceptable way for the neoliberal subject to fulfill his/her duty to consume as part of cycles of production and consumption. The remainder of this chapter will explore the way people consume alcohol as 'release', and how painkillers are used as part of this process. The combination of alcohol and analgesic medications to 'get more drunk' is a key example. The use of pain medications to quickly or more effectively return to a productive state after heavy alcohol use will also be explored.

Getting More Drunk

Majority of the participants in this study used alcohol to unwind after a busy week, and some spoke about using painkillers to enhance their experience with alcohol. Combining alcohol with painkillers is described as an enterprising way to enhance intoxication without having to resort to the expense of purchasing more alcohol or the difficulties around acquiring illicit drugs. Accounts of concurrent alcohol and analgesic use involve similar narratives to those produced by the young people who use illicit drugs, which were developed in Chapter 5: painkillers are presented as a convenient, commonplace product that can be drawn upon to manage or enhance experiences of intoxication. In this section however, the licit status of both alcohol and analgesic medications produces its own kind of legitimizing discourse among participants. An interview with a participant named 'Elizabeth' highlights some of the similarities, as well as difference, between participant discussion of illicit drug and alcohol use in combination with painkillers.

Elizabeth was born in Hong Kong, but has lived in Australia since she was a very small child. At the age of 32, Elizabeth now works a demanding job at a marketing company. Despite brief mention of being "*snowed under at work*" Elizabeth was not interested in talking about her job. She was, however, quite comfortable sharing vivid accounts of binge drinking and other forms of intoxication, which seemed to form a regular part of how she spent her weekends and other leisure time. Most of the discussion with Elizabeth surrounded recreational drug use, including alcohol, and painkillers. In a very plain speaking manner Elizabeth declares that she enjoys "*being messed up*", but only "*in the right setting. Obviously I wouldn't enjoy it if I was at work*".

Elizabeth goes on to explain that she does not find pleasure in using painkillers in a professional setting because when taking them, as she put it, "*I can't concentrate. I can't really function. I can't really think straight*". This loss of functionality is only desirable in the context of a night out:

> Like many people probably won't wonna dance until they're a bit more drunk or a bit more messed up. So I feel like I can enjoy friend's company a bit more. Especially if they are all high on illegal substances and they're all having conversations that are not that entertaining. It makes me more inclined to find it a bit more entertaining.

Here Elizabeth described a general context of casual night-time enjoyment, which is likely to involve licit and illicit drug use among herself and her friends. Painkillers are one of the substances she uses to get a "*buzz*", which she described as "*feel[ing] kind of like dizzy and light headed. Kind of like when I'm on other recreational drugs*".

Yet much of Elizabeth's discussion of analgesic use was when mixed with alcohol. She described several examples when out with friends who had taken ecstasy, but she either could not afford to join them or simply did not want to use illicit drugs that night. Elizabeth recalled one night when combining Panadeine Forte® and alcohol in place of ecstasy:

> It was my friend's birthday and they we're all taking [ecstasy] pills. And we went out to a club on Oxford St… I wasn't really feeling up for going out, and otherwise I would have just headed home. And I didn't even drink that much that night after taking them [Panadeine Forte®]. We [ended up being] out until six in the morning just dancing.

This became a common trope: "*So basically I just usually use them when I'm out in a pub drinking or something… I would just take like two Panadols® or I'd take like even a Panadeine Forte®, and I'd feel a bit of a buzz*". Through the combination of painkillers and alcohol Elizabeth could more easily, and cheaply, enjoy dancing and having "*silly conversations*" with friends, because it constituted a controlled loss of the control that operates in her everyday life. The night out is after all where, as she puts it, "*I'm meant to [be] doing that sort of stuff*". Painkillers like Panadeine Forte® and Panadol® also provide the opportunity to feel intoxicated without the risks associated with being very drunk. For Elizabeth, intoxication is the goal and painkillers were simply a "*cheaper way… to get more drunk*".

A framework around alcohol and painkillers being used to be more sociable also emerged from an interview with a participant who sought 'release' from periods of intense study. 'Henry' is a talkative 25-year-old who is an Arts graduate from a prestigious University. Tertiary education was a defining period for Henry, who described it with nothing but fondness. As a self-confessed more-awkward-than-most teenager, University was where Henry came into his own. Many of his enduring friendships were made during his time. Closely related to the social aspects of his time at University was the way in which friendships were forged through a joint commitment to periods of productive study and subsequent release: "*When I was studying for Uni I found that I really wanted to go out on the weekend because it's kind of Monday to Friday and Sunday that I did my study and I wanted to be able to have a bit of a break*".

Perhaps typical of University-educated men in their mid-twenties, Henry had a nonchalant attitude to intoxication and pleasure seeking through drug consumption. This was most clearly articulated when Henry spoke about drunken nights and drugged out adventures "*back in my Uni days*". Having seen his sister lose her life to heroin, Henry was, however, careful to mention that he had only occasionally taken illicit drugs, "*just experimentally and stuff*".

Recent debates about how best to describe periods of intense drinking on the weekend have provided critical theoretical accounts, as well as empirical evidence for, the conceptualization of this type of consumption as a form of 'calculated hedonism' (Szmigin et al. 2008). This involves patterns of measured but intense consumption that allow for a sense of controlled loss of control (Measham and Brain 2005). Henry's approach to drinking and drug use can be partly explained by this kind of purposeful and directed binge consumption that remains contained to very particular conditions, such as after the completion of his examinations and only with friends who have also completed similar milestone assessments.

During his University days, Henry also frequently mixed alcohol and painkillers because, as he puts it, "*you get drunk a lot faster*". He recalled one night when he went out to celebrate finishing his exams at a local bar: "*It's about 15-20 min' walk from the university… We went out and played some pool, listened to some music. They had some pretty cool computer games as well*". Described as a fairly standard night at the "*Uni bar*" Henry recalled:

> [I] had about 12 drinks that night. There were about eight of us there from different years from Uni. Different subjects as well. After we got to the bar we kind of broke up into three different sections. A few people played pool and a few people hung around the bar. I kind of jumped back and forth and in between.

After discovering a sheet of Nurofen Plus® that he had left in the pocket of his pants, Henry and his friend 'John' decided to take a few with their next drink.

Reflecting on his decision to take the Nurofen Plus® while drinking Henry said "*it wasn't illegal what we were doing. But I suppose it was the sense that maybe we were doing something morally or ethically which was a bit left of center and it might have been frowned upon*". However, when it came to painkillers Henry found comfort in the way the product was made, saying that painkillers are "*a quality product, by a quality pharmaceutical company. Similar thing with the alcohol as well*". His description here clearly represented an extension of the notion that painkillers are 'safe', but he goes further, blurring the line between the kinds of practices that they are safe for: "*I've drank alcohol before. I've had Panadol® before. Surely it wouldn't hurt that much by combining the two*". While combining alcohol and analgesics may attract some transgressive appeal, his use of these licit products was largely about enhancing an entirely normalized social practice: "*I was using them to get more drunk*".

A wide range of participants, including those introduced in the previous chapter, also mixed alcohol with painkillers. Heidi (27-year-old female) used to combine alcohol and painkillers when she was younger: "*[its] like being drunk, but better*". She says that she often used painkillers in this way on a Friday night after work, explaining that "*alcohol is a lot more expensive*" and that "*painkillers make a good alternative to just buying heaps of drinks*". Sean (26-year-old male), also introduced in Chapter 5, said that when mixing painkillers and alcohol "*you get drunk quick*". He recalled that the effect of the painkillers is different when taken with alcohol: "*it's not so much a painkilling effect, it's just that the drink is more effective. So you have a glass and you feel like you've had three*". This was described as a particularly good way to relax and enjoy the weekend: "*Things are good, you get chatty, and you loosen up. 'Cause it can be awkward if you're out socializing*".

The examples presented here demonstrate how practices of 'controlled consumption' for pleasurable release are often produced in response to periods of productive restraint. Elizabeth, for instance, specifies that "*being messed up*" is inappropriate for work and that periods of 'time out' are when she is supposed to "*do that sort of stuff*". Similarly,

Henry notes a distinct ritual of alcohol (and painkiller) consumption in response to periods of productive study. Other participants who use painkillers in combination with both illicit drugs and alcohol also provide important insight into the desire to engage in a form of 'controlled release'. There is, however, more to the combination of alcohol and painkillers than notions of release. Painkillers are not simply another way to become intoxicated. When compared to illicit drug use, painkillers are better suited to legitimate frameworks of personal consumption for pleasure.

Mixing painkillers with alcohol is seen as an acceleration of the effects of alcohol without the expense of increased alcohol consumption. The knowledge that painkillers are manufactured 'safely' is also an important driver of non-medical consumption with alcohol. Both products are seen as sanitary and thus in many ways safe, at least in comparison with illicit drugs. For those who make comparisons to illicit consumption, there is also an extra layer of personal, legal safety attributed to painkiller use. Painkillers are more commonplace than illicit drugs, and as such they are more available, and safer to acquire and possess.

Hangover Cure

The use of painkillers to relieve the symptoms of a hangover was also a significant point discussed among participants. The example of the hangover provides an important insight into the way periods of productive work and recreational play are connected; how they form part of the same cycle of restraint and release. Thus far, this chapter has discussed the use of painkillers to manage productive performance and to enhance periods of 'time out'. It is, however, significant to recognize that periods of productivity and release both form part of broader experiences of everyday life. Forms of self-medication for discomfort resulting from heavy alcohol consumption play an important part in the social organization of people's lives. While the pursuit of pleasurable intoxication is a common and expected part of the way participants took time out, they also required quick recovery from heavy alcohol (and other drug) use in order to be able to continue to function productively.

For some participants who use painkillers to remain productive, these medications also provided an easy opportunity to relieve hangovers. Michael, who was introduced earlier as someone who uses painkiller to 'bulldoze through' at work, also mentions incorporating analgesic consumption into his routine when drinking. When recalling what he does while drinking, Michael said:

> So I'm drinking and I'll do a preventative, so I know I'm not going to get it. 'Cause I'm a shocking hangover person and shocking headache person. So a lot of preventative taking. Sometimes I think "oh I'm going to get a headache or hangover" - who knows if I was or wasn't.

The kind of preventative use he describes when anticipating the symptoms of a headache at work are extended to the way he manages hangovers.

The use of painkillers for hangover pain also raises interesting questions about what constitutes medical use of an analgesic. While using painkillers for headache pain is common, participants did not always speak about the practice within a framework of legitimate medical consumption. For instance, Sarah often used a prescription painkiller to provide quicker relief from a hangover than an over-the-counter medication may have provided. She recalls one time when she had a bad hangover, saying "*I probably didn't need to take a prescription one but mum had it left over and my friend told me like if you take the Mersyndol Forte® then it will get rid of [the hangover] completely*". This worked well for Sarah as she could get on with her day quicker and get back to domestic work more easily: "*yeah it was good I could just get on with it and I did the washing and took the kids out as well*".

During an interview with Collin (25-year-old male), he explored the way experiences of pleasure can complicate medical consumption. When talking about the use of over-the-counter medications after periods of recreational (including licit and illicit) drug use, he explained that use of Panadol® for "*a hangover is not really medical, because it's something you brought on yourself*". Collin goes on to explain that analgesic use for headache pain blurs the line between medical and non-medical consumption. He is confident that people can reasonably manage their own use of the medication when headache and other pain occur: "*So if you know you've got reasonable pain and you know that what's gonna help is Panadeine Forte®, I'd say that's taking it for a medical reason*". Yet this kind of "*self-prescribing*" is also informed by medical notions of 'proper conduct' and 'responsible consumption':

> It's kind of a tipping point, it's half medical half recreational. 'Cause you bought it on yourself, but you are feeling like shit. And if you take a Panadol® when you've got a hangover you feel better.

Collin described medicine as a kind of omniscient moral arbiter that discourages heavy use of alcohol but is obliged to treat its consequences none-the-less: "*So it's medical, but the original medical condition is caused by recreational use of something else, like alcohol or whatever*".

Sean (26-year-old male) also discussed notions of pleasure in relation to painkiller use for hangovers. As well as the benefits of being able to recover from the hangover, Sean explained that he also enjoyed the physical sensation of the painkiller "*rejuvenating or healing*" his body. When describing the use of painkillers the morning after alcohol use, Sean says:

> You'll go out, and you'll be doing breakfast with the people you went out with the night before. Recapping. Debriefing. And someone will be like "hey hey, I've got some Nurofen Plus®" or "Panadeine Forte®". And you're just like "yes, I'm getting involved in that". Sit around and have it with your coffee and enjoy the slow release of pharmaceutical genius.

The "*pharmaceutical genius*" to which Sean is referring involved both the painkiller's ability to help him recover as well as the pleasurable sensation provided by its analgesic effects.

Accounts of painkiller consumption as "*hangover cure*" (Sarah) demonstrate how cycles of restraint and release are connected. The hangover is a physical state that lies between productivity and pleasure. The use of painkillers to alleviate this state can be part of a desire to return to productivity, to purge the body of the excesses of pleasure, or indeed form a pleasurable experience in-and-of itself.

Conclusion

This chapter has explored contemporary forms of work and play. It has elaborated on how neoliberal discourse has affected changes in modern working conditions, and how painkillers are used to achieve the ideals of flexibility and endurance through uncertainty endorsed by such discourse. A range of empirical examples demonstrate how participants use painkillers to 'bulldoze through' and 'deal with stress' at work, as well as to 'manage sleep' during busy periods of work. Use of painkillers to improve productive capacity is also extended to less traditional forms of work, such as helping to 'concentrate while studying' and 'taking care of the kids'. The therapeutic capacity of the painkiller is appropriated by individual consumers to pre-empt discomfort or illness likely to interrupt periods of productive work.

The requirement to be productive is also connected to the way participants engaged in 'time out'. Painkillers are used as a relatively safe and comparatively inexpensive way to 'get more drunk'. Comparisons to the normalization of illicit drug use are salient; however, this kind of consumption relates to broader time-out rituals that are embedded in the 'legitimate' economic and social order. The use of painkillers as a 'hangover cure' is also a key example of how productivity and release are connected. Using painkillers to accelerate recovery from a hangover allows participants to return to productive work sooner than they might otherwise have been able to.

Participants in this chapter describe how the ability to both 'work hard' and 'play hard' can be fostered or enhanced with the use of pain medications. While modern work and recreation have long been mediated by drugs, this chapter has argued that the conditions of late-modernity may permissively encourage individualized negotiations of health and consumer discourse in the pursuit of productive work and recreational release.

The next chapter will also explore the intersections of pleasure and health, this time in the context of chronic pain. It will elaborate on the significance of individual understandings of pain, the stigma attached to the chronic condition, and the associations of 'addiction' that haunt its treatment.

References

Åkerstedt, T., Knutsson, A., Westerholm, P., Theorell, T., Alfredsson, L., & Kecklund, G. (2002). Sleep Disturbances, Work Stress and Work Hours: A Cross-Sectional Study. *Journal of Psychosomatic Research, 53*(3), 741–748.

Australian Institute of Criminology. (2009). *Key Issues in Alcohol-Related Violence Research in Practice* (Summary Paper No. 4).

Baily, M. N., & Lawrence, R. (2001). Do We Have a New E-Conomy? (Working Paper 8243). National Bureau of Economic Research.

Barbieri, P. (2009). Flexible Employment and Inequality in Europe. *European Sociological Review, 25*(6), 621–628.

Bauman, Z. (2007). *Liquid Times: Living in an Age of Uncertainty*. Hoboken: Wiley.

Brain, K. (2000). *Youth, Alcohol, and the Emergence of the Post-Modern Alcohol Order*. London: Institute of Alcohol Studies.

Chatzitheochari, S., & Arber, S. (2009). Lack of Sleep, Work and the Long Hours Culture: Evidence from the UK Time Use Survey. *Work, Employment & Society, 23*(1), 30–48.

Clarke, A. E., Shim, J. K., Mamo, L., Fosket, J. R., & Fishman, J. R. (2003). Biomedicalization: Technoscientific Transformations of Health, Illness, and US Biomedicine. *American Sociological Review, 68*(2), 161–194.

Conrad, P., & Schneider, J. W. (1992). *Deviance and Medicalization: From Badness to Sickness*. Philadelphia: Temple University Press.

Cooper, M. (2008). *Life as Surplus: Biotechnology and Capitalism in the Neoliberal Era*. Seattle: University of Washington Press.

Duff, C. (2003). Drugs and Youth Cultures: Is Australia Experiencing the 'Normalization' of Adolescent Drug Use? *Journal of Youth Studies, 6*(4), 433–446.

Duff, C. (2005). Party Drugs and Party People: Examining the 'Normalization' of Recreational Drug Use in Melbourne. *Australia. International Journal of Drug Policy, 16*(3), 161–170.

Fazio, A., Joe-Laidler, K., Moloney, M., & Hunt, G. (2010). Gender, Sexuality, and Ethnicity as Factors of Club-Drug Use Among Asian Americans. *Journal of Drug Issues, 40*(2), 405–432.

Filmore, K. M., & Roizen, R. (2000). The New Manichaeism in Alcohol Science. *Addiction, 95*(2), 188–189.

Fortney, J., Curran, S., Fortney, G., Xiaotong, S., Booth, H., & Mukherjee, B. (2004). Factors Associated with Perceived Stigma for Alcohol Use and Treatment Among at-Risk Drinkers. *Journal of Behavioral Health Services & Research, 31*(4), 418–429.

Freeman, R. B. (2002). The Labour Market in the New Information Economy. *Oxford Review of Economic Policy, 18*(3), 288–305.

Gregg, M. (2011). *Work's Intimacy.* Hoboken: Wiley.

Harkness, A. M. B., Long, B. C., Bermbach, N., Patterson, K., Jordan, S., & Kahn, H. (2005). Talking About Work Stress: Discourse Analysis and Implications for Stress Interventions. *Work & Stress, 19*(2), 121–136.

Harrison, L., Kelly, P., Lindsay, J., Advocat, J., & Hickey, C. (2011). 'I Don't Know Anyone that Has Two Drinks a Day': Young People, Alcohol and the Government of Pleasure. *Health, Risk & Society, 13*(5), 469–486.

Hobbs, D. (2003). *Bouncers: Violence and Governance in the Night-Time Economy*. Oxford: Oxford University Press on Demand.

Keane, H. (2011). Drugs that Work: Pharmaceuticals and Performance Self-Management. In S. Fraser, & D. Moore (Eds.), *The Drug Effect: Health, Crime and Society*. Cambridge: Cambridge University Press.

McCreanor, T., Greenaway, A., Moewaka Barnes, H., Borell, S., & Gregory, A. (2005). Youth Identity Formation and Contemporary Alcohol Marketing. *Critical Public Health, 15*(3), 251–262.

Measham, F., & Brain, K. (2005). 'Binge' Drinking, British Alcohol Policy and the New Culture of Intoxication.*Crime, Media, Culture, 1*(3), 262–283.

Miller, P., Pennay, A., Jenkinson, R., Droste, N., Chikritzhs, T., Tomsen, S., et al. (2013). Patron Offending and Intoxication in Night Time Entertainment Districts (POINTED): A Study Protocol. *International Journal of Alcohol and Drug Research, 2*(1), 69–76.

Palley, T. I. (2005). From Keynesianism to Neoliberalism: Shifting Paradigms in Economics. In D. A. Johnston & A. Saad-Filho (Eds.), *Neoliberalism: A Critical Reader*. London: Pluto Press.

Parham, D. (2012). *Australia's Productivity Growth Slump: Signs of Crisis, Adjustment or Both?* Visiting Researcher Paper, Productivity Commission, Australian Government.

Rose, N. (2009). *The Politics of Life Itself: Biomedicine, Power, and Subjectivity in the Twenty-First Century*. Princeton: Princeton University Press.

Room, R. (2005). Stigma, Social Inequality and Alcohol and Drug Use. *Drug and Alcohol Review, 24*(2), 143–155.

Sanders, B. (2012). Gang Youth, Substance Use Patterns, and Drug Normalization. *Journal of Youth Studies, 15*(8), 1–17.

Shacham, E., & Cottler, L. (2010). Sexual Behaviors Among Club Drug Users: Prevalence and Reliability. *Archives of Sexual Behavior, 39*(6), 1331–1341.

Smith, P., & Morton, G. (2006). Nine Years of New Labour: Neoliberalism and Workers' Rights. *British Journal of Industrial Relations, 44*(3), 401–420.

Steptoe, A., Peacey, V., & Wardle, J. (2006). Sleep Duration and Health in Young Adults. *Archives of Internal Medicine, 166*(16), 1689–1692.

Szmigin, I., Griffin, C., Mistral, W., Bengry-Howell, A., Weale, L., & Hackley, C. (2008). Re-framing 'Binge Drinking' as Calculated Hedonism: Empirical Evidence from the UK. *International Journal of Drug Policy, 19*(5), 359–366.

Tomsen, S. (2003). Bouncers: Violence and Governance in the Night-time Economy. *Current Issues in Criminal Justice, 15*(2), 200.

Tomsen, S., Homel, R., & Thommeny, J. (1990). *Situational Factors in Alcohol-Related Public Assaults*. National Committee on Violence/National Drug Offensive.

Wainwright, D., & Calnan, M. (2000). Rethinking the Work Stress 'Epidemic'. *The European Journal of Public Health, 10*(3), 231–233.

7

Chronic Pain and Dependence: Chronic Conditions, Opiates and Stigma

Chronic pain is a debilitating condition that can have a range of serious consequences on the lives of those who experience it. The kind of constant suffering experienced by people with chronic pain can interfere with their ability to work or participate in social activities. While an initial injury or condition is often identifiable as the original source of pain, medical knowledge is limited in its capacity to explain why such pain is ongoing (DePalma et al. 2011). The frustration that accompanies an inability to fully participate in work or social activities, and a lack of knowledge about why, is also detrimental to the mental and emotional health of those who experience chronic pain (Dow et al. 2012). Indeed, epidemiological research has made strong links between chronic pain and the development of clinical forms of depression and anxiety (Bair et al. 2008; Gureje et al. 1998; Fishbain et al. 1997).

Another important aspect of the experience of chronic pain that contributes to the emotional difficulties that accompany it, is the stigma associated with both the condition and its treatment. Chapter 4's discussion of medical approaches to pain already established that the chronic pain patient is subject to stigma, including from within the medical profession. At the 2010 Pain Summit, which was a gathering

G. C. Dertadian, *A Fine Line*,
https://doi.org/10.1007/978-981-13-1975-4_7

of pain medicine professionals experts, a reduction in the stigma associated with chronic pain was named as a priority for the specialty of pain medicine (2010). The treatment of chronic pain often involves regular and ongoing use of pharmaceutical opiates. The conflation of regular pharmaceutical opiates use with illicit and 'addictive' opiate consumption is an important aspect of the stigmatization and marginalization of the chronic pain patient.

This chapter will explore three empirical examples that illustrate different aspects of the relationship between pain, chronic conditions and drug dependence. It begins by discussing tensions within the medical profession about how to treat pain, which help to frame the discussion that follows. The chapter then focuses primarily on the lives and experiences of two participants, who will be referred to as 'Allan' and 'Mark', both of whom suffer from chronic physical pain. The chapter discusses how chronic pain has affected their lives, and the way they consume analgesic medications. It addresses the two men's experiences of stigma and discusses their understanding of problematic and dependent painkiller use. Finally, the chapter explores the life of a participant named 'Jake', who has experienced chronic emotional pain and who has become dependent on opiates as a result. This chapter explores the way chronic pain affects the lives of those who experience it by providing an in-depth exploration of three different life histories. Some of the details of the lives of these men have been altered to ensure anonymity.

Treating Chronic Pain

Before embarking on an exploration of the lives of Allan, Mark and Jake, it is useful to revisit medical approaches to analgesic use for the treatment of chronic pain. Chapter 4 has already outlined the way medical approaches to opiates use vary across different medical fields and their associated literatures. Of note was the biopsychosocial model endorsed by the specialty of pain medicine. This approached advocates for a model of care that incorporates clinical observation of the patient's psychological and social well-being alongside more traditional forms of biological assessment. The use of opiate analgesics is still a significant component of the treatment programs recommended under the biopsychosocial model. Advocacy for reducing the stigmatization of the chronic pain patient is also a notable feature of pain medicine literature (Cohen et al. 2011; Holloway et al. 2007).

There is, however, a distinct tension between the pain medicine literature's advocacy for a biopsychosocial approach and the prevalence of more traditional biomedical forms of medical training. The limited capacity for medical practitioners to independently verify a treatable pathology in many chronic pain patients contributes to the stigmatization of pain patients (Cohen et al. 2011). Sections of the pain medicine literature acknowledge that physicians are often left with a limited framework for understanding pain outside of a biomedical model and thus can become frustrated with and distrusting of the chronic pain patient (Macrae 2001; Thomas 2000; McCaffery and Thorpe 1989). Reliance on the subjective evaluations of the client's experiences of pain may also cause tension in a relationship typically controlled by the medical professional (Lupton 2012: 113). Exchanges about pain interrupt established power differentials between the doctor and the patient by placing the patient's subjective experience of bodily discomfort over the doctor's expertise of the body. In general, practice in particular chronic pain is thus often dismissed as either being psychosomatically produced or not traditionally treatable (Cohen et al. 2011).

Chronic pain patients are particularly vulnerable to stigma if they consume opiates, leading to a perception in the medical profession that they already behave like 'drug addicts'. One Norwegian study has, for instance, noted that, for women in particular, pain patients feel the need to attempt "to fit in with normative, biomedical expectations of correctness" and that it is "hard work behaving as a credible patient" (Werner and Malterud 2003: 1409). An anthropological study at a US Veterans Affairs clinic has described the ambivalence of medical practitioners toward the pain patient. The study observes that there is a prevalent assumption among physicians that requests for medical prescriptions are equivalent to drug seeking: an article published from the study is aptly titled "No one wants to be the candy man" (Crowley-Matoka and True 2012). This is also complicated by the heightened political context surrounding the prescription of opiates, for which some US prescribers have even been charged with criminal offences (Reidenberg and Willis 2007).

This section has developed a series of observations about the treatment of chronic pain within the medical profession. It has outlined how tensions within the medical perspective about how to treat the pain patient and pejorative comparisons to drug dependence inform the stigmatization of chronic pain. All of these tensions play out in various ways in the lives of three participants who have had very different encounters with chronic pain, stigma and medication consumption. The remainder of the chapter explores the life histories of Allan, Mark and Jake.

Two Patients, Two Stories

This section will introduce two participants in this study who have experienced chronic pain: Allan and Mark. It provides a brief exploration of how they developed chronic pain and explains the role analgesic and other opiates play in their treatment and beyond. This section introduces these men and their experiences of chronic pain and pain relief before the rest of the chapter explores these issues in more detail.

In 1999, at the age of 32, Allan was a married man and father of a 3-year-old son with special needs. The family lived in a small suburban home in North-West Sydney, in an area best known as the 'bible belt' of the city. Allan worked a stable job for a government agency to support his family as well as to pay for the treatment required for his son's condition. In early 1999, Allan was involved in a workplace accident that resulted in an injury to his back and ongoing chronic pain: "*I did my back in. Prolapsed disc. But it didn't stop there*". He was prescribed a range of high-dose opiate analgesics to help with the pain.

Months after sustaining the injury Allan was still unable to work: "*I was in pain. It was excruciating. I couldn't do anything*". Allan and the family soon began to consider surgical interventions to help alleviate ongoing chronic pain. After receiving advice from two different specialists it became clear that the surgery, which centered on delicate areas of the lower back and spine, had its risks. Allan agonized over the decision, and even asked the surgeon "*if it were you, would you do the surgery?*" Allen brought his father, a pharmacist, for support in the final consultation: "*When it was time to make a decision as to whether or not to have this back operation after the first injury, I took my father with me, who is one of the most clear thinking guys I've ever met*". He was booked in for surgery the very next week.

Three months after the operation Allan returned to work. His job involves coordinating human and technical resources and describes it as such: "*my job is just a little bit short of life threatening - I mean we could make mistakes and people might get hurt... and yeah you need to have your faculties about you*". He recalled that the medications he was being prescribed after the surgery (OxyContin® and Endone®) sometimes impacted his ability to work: "*I reflected a couple of times on just the medication alone prevented me from working*". This meant that he mostly preferred low dose medications that allowed him to be "*clearheaded*".

Ongoing pain and continued interruptions to work made Allen's employment more precarious over the next few years, and in 2001 Allan decided to undergo another surgical intervention. The operation was successful and Allan's pain was temporarily reduced. However, in 2006 Allan experienced a relapse of his injury for which he entered a private hospital for pain management. It was during his time in hospital and just after release that Allan most commonly used prescription opiates: "*straight after the morphine, straight after the operation and then straight after the flare ups again they've given me those ones [OxyContin®]*". Allan says that he would move as quickly as possible to lower-dose medications because he did not like how it felt being on high-dose opiates: "*just not being able to operate, that was the opiate... the sheer unstraight-headedness that it was causing*". Still, the prescription medications were essential to getting him back on his feet after relapse.

Six months prior to interview, Allan experienced another injury relapse, leaving him only able to work part-time. His wife also fell ill around the same time and his son's doctors indicated that they were concerned about how the pair were going to be able to manage (and afford) her care. Feeling overwhelmed, Allan reflects: "*A couple of problems [have] come at once, which makes care harder, care for our son harder, which in turn adds to the stress and then, it's just a vicious circle isn't it*".

Mark is another participant who has experienced problems with chronic pain. His life trajectory, however, took a different path to that of Allan's. In 1987, Mark was a working-class 25-year-old tradesman. Enjoying the flexibility of not having to work full time for a large company, Mark was mostly employed on short-term contracts. One night in May of 1987, after an uncomfortable evening of disrupted sleep, he was hospitalized for osteomyelitis of the spine. Osteomyelitis is an infection of the bone that is known to be painful (Collert 1977; Zimmerli 2010). Mark recalls: "*It debilitates you so you can't walk. And it works in the spine so its really painful, so I had to have a lot of pain medication*". He remained hospitalized for a period of approximately 6 months, where he was on a regular dose of morphine.

As the osteomyelitis began to improve Mark was released as an outpatient to a team of pain specialists that prescribed OxyContin®. After approximately one month, the pain team began to taper down Mark's dose of OxyContin®: "*the pain team they always rely on that, 'oh well we've got to start weening you off the Oxys and put you onto this lower drugs'*". Still experiencing serious pain for months after being released from hospital, Mark became increasingly frustrated by the pain team's approach. Though his pain had become "*much better*", it often flared up unexpectedly. The unpredictability of Mark's pain had a debilitating effect on his ability to work. Without a prescribed dose of an appropriate opiate, Mark became unwilling to commit to large or long-term contracts.

In order to manage the unpredictable pain and to provide some stability in his work, Mark started to acquire OxyContin® from an inner-city "*dealer*" on a regular basis: "*I remember when I legitimately had a lot of pain, they wanted to take me off the painkillers. So I couldn't sleep or work or anything like that. So I felt like I had no choice*". By October of 1989, Mark had been taking opiates on an ongoing basis for approximately 16 months, which at this point had mostly been prescribed to him by a physician in relation to his osteomyelitis and ongoing chronic pain. As a result, his level of tolerance was so high that the oral ingestion of opiates had little effect anymore. Desperate to be able to work and live without the pain, Mark turned to intravenous and heroin use.

At the time of interview, Mark had spent the best part of the previous 25 years living 'on the street' and injecting drugs. He reflects on his life since the original hospitalization with a deep sense of despair: "*I'm living this illegal sort of underground life-style. I mean how can you esteem yourself? You're not working. You've got no goals. You have nothing stimulating to wake up to everyday*". The years between Mark's injury and the interview will be explored in the sections that follow.

Living with Chronic Pain

One important element of the trajectories of the lives of Allan and Mark is the way chronic pain has affected their life circumstances. Constant pain and heavy reliance on pain medications produced a range of difficult circumstances that required or initiated changes to their lives. As noted above, Allan's ability to attend work and perform his role effectively has been drastically compromised for significant periods over the last 15 years. Over the years, Allan's position at work has become increasingly uncertain and, six months prior to interview he was forced to move to a part-time position. This had a significant negative impact on the family's financial situation.

Impact on work was not, however, the only way chronic pain effected Allan's life. He is also a passionate volunteer for a community safety organization: "*I've been a volunteer for 29 and a half years, since I was sixteen. And I love caring for the community*". Prior to his injury, Allan was heavily involved in volunteer rescue and support operations in the organization. An inability to perform the physical tasks required for this kind of involvement meant that Allan's role in the community organization was significantly diminished after his injury: "*my ability to carry out most of my function within that organization was completely damaged at the same time that I had my operation, or my injury*". Given the unpredictability of his condition, and the fact that rescue and support operations occasionally involved people whose lives are in danger, Allan decided that he would have to find other ways to be involved in the organization: "*I've found some other ways to use my skills, I do a lot more training now instead of operating than I used to*". His role in training has, however, been much less fulfilling.

Chronic pain also impacts Allan's ability to care for his son, who has a behavioral disorder. Aside from his capacity to work and thus finance various treatments, pain also limits Allan's ability to, for instance, help his son get dressed in the morning or get him to the doctor: "*sometimes I just kind of feel useless, and that can be really stressful*". At the time of interview Allan's son had been hospitalized for six weeks, and a recent flare up meant he was not able to visit as often as he would like.

Discussion about care for his son also sparked reflection on the connection between stress and health: "*I think the body is so intertwined. How injury can cause stress and how stress can cause injury*". He described an intimate relationship between the stresses associated with the deteriorating health of his wife and son and his own health:

> My wife and I are very conscious that my son's problems have been at their worse for the last three years, and just in the last year or so my wife's health hasn't been well either. Where the doctors used to say "be careful of your health because, if you deteriorate, your care deteriorates". That's sort of come to pass now.

Allan goes on to explain that his most recent flare up may have had a lot to do with stress about the family's health:

> Because my back went twice, [in the past] I could pinpoint the injury. Whereas this time I hadn't had any [physical activity] - I wasn't in the cubical trying on clothes and got up the wrong way. I've got nothing to point to this time… That's one thing that's freaked me out, that perhaps my flare up this time was more to do with [worrying about] my son than [my] actual injury.

Beyond the physical debilitation of chronic pain, stress forms a significant element of the way chronic pain affects Allan's life, his ability to work and care for his family. Allan's observations about the relationship between stress and physical health are salient examples of why the biopsychosocial model has emerged in medical discourse.

For Mark, living with chronic pain is inseparable from the use of pain medications. Mark explains that, after his injury he spent a long time in hospital and opiate use was a mundane part of that experience. After leaving the hospital, Mark's pain team provided instructions about how and when to use his medications. He goes on to explain that even when not prescribed to him directly, for many years his use of OxyContin® was in line with the instructions that physicians had provided: "*I was just doing what the doctors had told me to do*".

As Mark began to obtain OxyContin® from street-based drug markets, the pain team became increasingly suspicious of how he was acquiring his medications and eventually stopped prescribing them altogether. His pain specialist moved him onto lower-dose over-the-counter analgesics such as Panadeine Extra® and Nurofen® that did not satisfactorily cover the pain: "*but I was still in pain, I still needed to work, so I had to continue using [opiates]*". Not knowing when the pain would return, and not having access to an appropriate dose of analgesic to manage it, made contractual commitments to physical labor difficult. This was the primary reason for Mark's initial use of heroin. On the recommendation of a long-term friend who had been helping him acquire OxyContin®, Mark decided to inject heroin to properly ameliorate the pain of a particularly nasty flare up while in the middle of an important job.

Within the context of persistent physical pain that was producing instability in his employment, Mark decided to manage the situation as best he could: "*So I was forced, through the pain, to go and get the drugs off the street*". For approximately 6 months following this initial injection of heroin Mark used both OxyContin® and heroin intravenously on an intermittent basis: "*[at the start] it didn't really affect my life as much as you might think*". However, as Mark became more and more immersed in the street culture of Kings Cross, where he "*scored*" (acquired) and "*banged up*" (injected) most of his drugs, intravenous consumption began to gather some pleasurable and emotional significance. Opiate injection became a respite from the pain, a kind of relief that had been rare since leaving hospital a few years earlier.

Using Opiates and Other Analgesics

Allan and Mark had different responses to and experiences with their medications. While Allan felt that, on balance, lower-dose medication provided a better outcome, Mark regarded over-the-counter analgesics to be entirely ineffective in reducing his pain. This section will elaborate on the two men's personal experiences using opiates and other analgesics. It explores the way analgesic medications form part of life routines and canvasses the meanings that have become attached to such consumption in their lives.

Allan's use of painkillers was largely restricted to over-the-counter analgesics, except during periods of unexpected flare up or relapse. His use of Panadeine Extra® is the most regular of all the medications he has used since the injury. Allan does not like using prescription opiates (such as OxyCOntin® and Endone®) and he limits their use to times when his pain is otherwise unbearable:

> They're about the only times I've used it, is straight after the morphine, straight after the operation and then straight after the flare ups again they've given me those ones. Yeah no literally the strongest thing I take is Panadeine Forte®

One of the main reasons for this is that Allan is unable to concentrate when using prescription medication such as OxyContin®. This is particularly problematic when at work, dealing with potential injuries in the community: "*it's just a realization that you know you probably could cause something to happen bad if you did try and work with that sort of level of non-clear-headedness*".

Still, Allan says that the use of high dose and prescription pain medications, including OxyContin®, is a vital part of his ability to perform everyday functions:

> at the end of the day I would be worse if I wasn't taking what I'm taking when I'm taking it. And to a certain degree I've got to be - it's the only way to really manage my day-to-day affairs when I'm at my worse.

Allan describes a complex relationship with his pain and prescription medications. While pharmaceutical opiates were selectively useful in getting Allan back on his feet after a flare up, they could be equally problematic by impairing his ability to think clearly.

For Mark, opiate use had different kinds of significance at different times in his life. For the first two years after his initial hospitalization, Mark was simply using opiates at the direction of his doctors. Opiates were a common part of his treatment: "*it felt like they gave them to me almost every day*". However, as the pain team tapered down Mark's dose and he began to obtain his OxyContin® via illicit means, acquiring the medication and using it became a necessary routine in order to stay in work: "*I was always trying to find more, just in case*". Once he transitioned to intravenous use of OxyContin® pleasure began to enter in the equation. After a year of intravenous use the line between pain relief and pleasurable inebriation had become indistinct for Mark: "*cause I was in pain but I also liked the way it made me feel*".

Mark spoke in detail about the euphoric feeling that opiates provided. He explains:

> They give you a really good feeling inside. They're a good relaxant. There's no side-effects psychologically. You know, you don't have any hallucinations or anything like that. You just feel a tremendous peace and a warmth.

In another vivid description of the way he feels when using opiates Mark compares the physical sensation of an opiate high to the Christian notion of the Holy Spirit:

> From a spiritual perspective, a lot of people have felt the Holy Spirit. And in their testimony in church they've said they felt a beautiful warmth come upon me. Well I liken the euphoric effect of painkillers to it being a FALSE [emphasis added] Holy Spirit, 'cause it feels like the Holy Spirit.

This feeling of a "*beautiful warmth*" is described as particularly appealing, and an important part of the reason why Mark continues to use opiates: "*that's why it's so desirable, why people want to experience it again and again and again. It becomes better than an orgasm you know*".

Mark has also used heroin—or 'gear'—interchangeably with pharmaceutical opiates over the last 20 years. While pharmaceutical opiates and heroin are described as "*pretty similar really*", Mark does emphasize the benefits of injecting prescribed opiates. He explains that: "*With the Oxys you're guaranteed that you know what you're getting. And it's very strong, 'cause it's legal. With the gear, it's Russian roulette. You don't know what you're getting*". While pharmaceutical opiates are regarded as safer and more ideal, sometimes heroin is all that is available: "*sometimes there's no Oxy on the street and so you go for the gear instead*". Occasionally Mark even prefers to inject heroin instead of OxyContin®: "*Just for a change. [If] I was told there was really good gear on the street. Really potent, really strong*".

The pain-relieving and pleasurable aspects of Mark's opiate use are also tied to the consequences of stigma associated with his dependence. Stigma had significant impact on how Mark felt about himself and thus his experiences of emotional pain, which he subsequently self-medicated with opiate use. Allan experienced stigma of a different kind, more closely associated with his chronic pain condition and how he used medications to treat it. The next section will discuss Allan and Mark's experiences of stigma and how they have dealt with it over the years.

Dealing with Stigma

Dealing with stigma was an important part of Allan and Mark's experiences of chronic pain and opiate use. The conditions they suffer from and the way they use analgesics to manage various forms of pain were a constant source of stigma. Sociological accounts of stigma indicate that the concept is a manifestation of the social disapproval of traits or behaviors that society deems to be outside the 'norm' (Goffman 1963). The way people experience stigma and internalize pronouncements of 'shame' has also been a key features of the sociology of stigma, particularly as it relates to chronic health conditions (Steward et al. 2008). The inability to objectively/medically verify pain and the often-ambiguous source of its chronic relapse inform its disapproval, weather consciously by a health care professional or structurally through the system in which they operate. Moreover, the moral weight attached to dependent and illicit consumption produces a range of marginalizing consequences for those experiencing or deemed to engaged in such consumption. Both Allan and Mark reflected on how types of social disapproval impact the way they live their lives.

Allan says that stigma often surrounds his inability to do basic everyday tasks properly when he is in pain. He explains that his family often do not understand how the pain affects his ability to function and do basic tasks:

> I even have trouble convincing my own family, my own wife that I'm in pain or I've got a problem or I need some help. So for example if I ask her if you wouldn't mind making me a cuppa [cup of tea] there's probably a reason, but she'll just roll her eyes.

Allan reflects that part of the problem is that his injury is not visible:

> My injury, my disability is very much an unseen - it's not a broken leg, I haven't got plaster on my arm… I just wish sometimes that I had a cast on my leg or my arm because people would know what we go through.

His use of medications also adds to this stigma:

> If I take that [box of medication] out and put it on my desk at work, which is my one day's medication type thing, morning, lunch, evening and night… if people see that at work… [they] think "you're a hypochondriac" - we often joke about how I keep the drug companies going because it's just my use alone. Yeah no there's an ostracization I believe just in that alone.

Allan expresses concern about what kind of impression his use of medications leaves on his co-workers. He wonders if they think "*is he a druggy because he's got all that?*" or "*is he any less of a worker because he's on that sort of a medication?*" Allan mostly tries to brush off these concerns with humor: "*I often joke about how I've got uppers and downers, and that ones to go with that ones *haha**".

Stigma and marginalization have also played a role in Mark's life over the last 25 years. Mark explains that the assumption that he is 'drug seeking' has eroded his relationship with the medical profession and those who have treated his chronic pain: "*as soon as they get it into their minds that you are abusing them they just stop caring, stop treating you properly*". He goes on to explain that, after feeling abandoned by his doctors and developing a regular pattern of opiate injecting, the stigma of intravenous use affected all of the relationships in his life: "*I'm ostracized from my family. I have no meaningful relationship with anybody anymore*". This kind of marginalization also has a detrimental impact of Mark's sense of self-worth:

> It's not just the painkillers, it's all the social problems that it brings. You know unemployment. And especially how it impacts on your confidence and self-esteem and how you feel about yourself. You know even though you can support your addiction and everything, it's nothing to be proud of. It just eats away at you.

In Mark's case the assumption of 'drug seeking', and the stigma associated with it, is implicated in his eventual development of problematic patterns of opiate use that have had a devastating impact on his life.

Mark felt a deep sense of suffering at the injustice of this stigma, even describing it as a form of pain: "*The torment that you go through from being addicted to painkillers and the tricks you have to do to sustain it… so you feel a lot of mental pain when that happens*". He goes on to explain that the only way he now has to escape the stigma and its impact on his life is to go to sleep. However, not having had stable housing for the past 10 years makes sleep an uncertainty. Part of the reason why he continues to inject pharmaceutical opiates and heroin is to help him get to sleep wherever and whenever he can: "*I mean I actually enjoy going to sleep, when I can. It's like a bit of a relief or release from the consciousness of the hell that I'm in. It turns it off. I escape just by being asleep*".

For both Allan and Mark, the stigma of chronic pain and drug use has had significant impacts of their lives. One important element of the stigma that surrounds chronic pain and analgesic use is its relationship to substance use and drug dependence. Concerns about the nature and definition of problematic and dependent consumption in the lives of Allan and Mark will be the subject of the next section.

Problematic and Dependent Consumption?

Concern about problematic and dependent consumption was often raised by Allen and Mark. Allan spoke about concerns regarding the way he uses his medications, though he was reluctant to describe these as 'addictive' behavior. While Mark raised a range of concerns about the use of pain medication, which he directly refers to as part of an 'addiction'. This section will compare the way the two participants define and experience problematic or dependent consumption of pain medications.

At the time of interview, Allan had been using pain medications "*pretty long-term and pretty seriously over the last 14 odd years*". This meant that Allan had had a long time to think about the complexity of how and why he uses pain medications. Allan remarks that:

> I've reflected to myself whether or not I should be taking a certain level of drugs or whether you get yourself into a false sense of, "if I take this pain-killer, is it going to prevent pain later or not".

Allan says that he often wonders whether his use is, what he refers to as "*proactive or reactive*". He goes on to explain that reactive use is in response to pain, and can thus be considered more legitimate: "*you know within yourself that if you're hurting you take a Panadol® and if you're hurting more you might need a Panadeine®*". The use of painkillers in response to pain was juxtaposed with the use of painkillers in anticipation of pain: Allan's 'proactive use'.

Allan engaged in proactive use to avoid the emergence of pain in order to make sure he could get a good night's sleep, or be able to function at work—comparison to the instrumental use described in the previous chapter is salient. He explains that he often takes painkillers before he goes to bed, whether in pain or not. This ensures that Allan will be able to sleep without worrying: "*The nights I forget to or don't take it [Panadol®], I know the night's not going to be as good. I'll have more broken sleep*". He also uses painkillers most days before work, so that he can avoid the possibility of a painful flare up: "*sometimes I know its gonna be a busy day and I just take them before the pain starts*".

Part of Allan's dilemma revolves around the idea that, while outside of the convention of his medical treatment, proactive use often makes his life much easier. Allan wonders how often he uses painkillers to allow for better sleep or to make his work bearable, rather than to more directly relieve pain. This also extends to his family life: "*I'm in a better position to deal with family life and home if I'm not quite in pain. I think I might function a bit better*". The ability to avoid pain, or to eliminate the possibility of it affecting his day is a significant part of how Allan now uses his pain medications: "*I'm sure that I operate better when I'm not in pain… and when I take a Panadol® I don't have to worry about it*". It is, however, this kind of painkiller use that stirs concern about the propriety of his consumption: "*am I doing the wrong thing by using them proactively?*"

Concern about whether proactive use is the "*wrong way to use painkillers*" also prompted comparisons to recreational and dependent consumption. While recalling one time at work when Allan had used a prescription painkiller proactively he said: "*It was quite a funky feeling obviously - I take it that that must be what recreational drug use would give you*". He was also quick to note "*I've never used a recreational drug in my life*". When explaining that he uses painkillers almost every day, and that he has been doing so for years Allan despairs that:

> You hear the saying that too much medication and for too long can be not good for your health and I always try to think how to reduce the amount. But to a certain degree with my disability it'll never - I'll never be tablet free again.

While his descriptions above imply a significant dependence on pain medications to function without pain, Allan went on to quickly dispel any implication that he was 'addicted': "*I don't class myself as being addicted to any form of medication*".

For Allan proactive use is aimed at making his day more efficient and easier to manage, yet concern about the appropriateness of his consumption illustrates how addiction discourse can encroach on practices of consumption. While Allan expressed concern about the 'wrong' way to use painkillers and a dependence on them to function without pain, a framework of 'addiction' was still excluded from his experience. For Allan, ongoing pain and the use of low dose analgesics provide a legitimizing framework that is not compatible with notions of 'addiction': "*I don't believe one five milligram tablet of paracetamol per day, neither does my doctor believe, that there is anything to be worried about*".

Unlike Allan, Mark often referred to his painkiller use as part of an 'addiction': he describes himself as being 'addicted' to pain medications and refers to himself as an 'addict'. Importantly however, it is not just the regular consumption of painkillers that defines addiction for Mark. Participation in illicit activities and the social marginalization that accompanies it are central to the way Mark experiences addiction. For instance, in order to maintain a level of financial stability, and to sustain his drug use, Mark sells drugs on a regular basis. Part way through the interview Mark fielded a call from a young woman who was looking to acquire ecstasy pills for the weekend. After finishing the call Mark says "*This is what keeps me afloat. You haven't got many other options when you're an addict*".

The way Mark acquires his medications is also significant to note. While Mark buys a portion of his OxyContin® from the illicit drug market, he also acquires a range of prescriptions from different physicians: "I*'ve got five doctors I go and see. Yeah well because of my history [with osteomyelitis] and everything I've got all of the documentation*". Mark is also sure to remain abreast of policy developments and how they might impact his ability to acquire opiates. When referring to policy discussion surrounding the electronic monitoring of pharmaceutical purchases, Mark says he has already prepared for its potential introduction by learning how to alter identification cards: "*It's very easy to go to an internet cafe and change the names and everything*". These forms of deceptive and criminal behavior are an important part of how Mark constitutes his experience as an 'addict':

> So they put all these little hurdles before us. But because the addiction is so strong, it's so powerful, you can get over it, get around it. But really it's just another trick of a lot of tricks you have to do when you're an addict.

It is not simply the regular use of pain medications or the injecting use of heroin that constitutes Mark's experience of addiction. Despite regular use of prescription opiates when in hospital and just following his release from hospital, Mark rarely referred to himself as an 'addict' during this time. However, his descriptions of the political economy of criminal activity required to sustain his drug use were replete with references to addiction.

Reflecting on his dependence and the way in which it required involvement in crime, Mark explained that he felt abandoned by the medical practitioners charged with his care. After his original hospitalization, medical staff prescribed him opiates for a period of 18 months. Once Mark was dependent on the medication, it was taken away and he was left in circumstances he felt unequipped to deal with: "*This all started… [from] being in hospital. And it's just been hell ever since. 'Cause it's a trap. You're in a trap you can't get out of*". While Mark acknowledges that chronic pain is not the only reason why he continues to use opiates, he defends against the stigma of a "*crazy drug fiend*" that he is often subject to:

> Initially I didn't voluntarily go out and use drugs for leisure or anything… I was on morphine, they prescribed me morphine because of osteomyelitis in the spine. And by the time I left the hospital I was hooked, I was dependent on the morphine. Part of the pain team management was Oxy, and that's how I got hooked on them.

He is also highly critical of the way the medical profession has dealt with his substance use: "*A lot of people say that people who are addicted are sick. You know it's an illness… so they should want to help you, but they just don't give a fuck*". In Mark's case, it is important to recognize that he did not have a previous medical history of substance use and that his medical care (or lack of it) is in fact a central turning point in his development of problematic consumption and 'addictive' behaviors.

The stigma associated with addiction has had debilitating effects on the conditions of Mark's life: "*It's just destroyed my life*". Living under the uncertain and criminalized conditions that characterize cultures of injecting drug use for more than 20 years has taken its toll:

> I've been addicted to them for years. Everything is focused on getting them, using them. And everything suffers. Relationships with family and friends. Especially relationships with yourself.

Mark's sense of self has been eroded by having to "*hustle for the basics*" for so long. Moreover, this lack of self-confidence is solidified by structural marginalization: "*I've got no education in order to get a decent job. So I've no access to credit or anything that can help to give sort of quality of lifestyle*". He is bleak and defeated as he reflects: "*using painkillers and addiction, it takes away all hope. So if you have no hope there's not much to look forward to at all*".

Chronic Emotional Pain?

It is clear from the examples discussed thus far that chronic physical pain brings with it changing life circumstances and forms of social stigma that are emotionally difficult. Allan felt ostracized from his work and family life and experienced a sense of loss at not being able to continue his lifelong participation with a community organization, as well as take care of his wife and son. Similarly, Mark felt betrayed by medical practitioners charged with his care. This was related to other forms of suffering as he was forced to live 'on the street' and engage in criminal activity. Allan and Mark's lives are salient examples of the significance of the emotional elements of pain. From these experiences, a series of related questions about emotional pain unrelated to physical injury also emerge as noteworthy. The remainder of this section explores the life of a third participant who has encountered prolonged periods of emotional pain and uses painkillers to alleviate it.

Jake was born in 1983 and was 29 at the time of interview. His family home is in the culturally diverse, though largely disadvantaged area of South-West Sydney. In 2000, at the age of 17, Jake was introduced to a young woman named 'Louise' through mutual friends. The pair fell in love hard and fast. After four years with Louise, she became the victim of a violent assault, which, after a short period of hospitalization, resulted in her death. Though the crime had occurred almost a decade before the interview, it still commands a great deal of Jake's emotional energy. Jake was unable to sleep for months after Louise's murder and he visited a range of community health services which "*were basically shit and didn't help at all*".

Jake was first introduced to OxyContin® by a friend a few months after Louise's death: "*I started using them to block that out because I couldn't sleep at night and a friend put me onto them and I was trying all sorts of other drugs just to knock myself out*". During this time, Jake also experimented with cocaine, amphetamines and benzodiazepines, among other drugs, to try and help cope with the loss.

Over a period of approximately 6 months, OxyContin® began to emerge as Jake's drug of choice. For a time, OxyContin® seemed to allow Jake some respite from the difficult emotions associated with the death of his girlfriend, and he gradually started to use the medication more frequently:

> I started out using maybe one pill a fortnight and I went to a pill a week and it got worse and started being nearly every day and eventually probably after about twelve months or so using got really addicted to them and couldn't basically start the day without one.

After appropriately 18 months, Jake noticed that his use of OxyContin® was becoming a problem, and he entered a local rehabilitation program in early 2007. He had a mixed response to his experience in the facility, but noted that "*at least I got off them for a while*".

Still struggling with feelings of loneliness Jake return to occasional oral OxyContin® use in May of 2007, but found that long periods of regular oral ingestion had rendered his tolerance high enough not to feel the effects very much anymore. In April of 2008, a friend who had been supplying Jake with OxyContin® recommended that he tried injecting methadone to "*get a good night's sleep*". Jake recalled "*I liked the feeling, the experience I had on it [methadone]*". Encouraged by the "*relaxing effect*", Jake's initial intravenous use of methadone was followed rapidly by a spate of intravenous heroin use:

> After a few weeks of using that I couldn't get methadone anymore so I got introduced to a heroin dealer and started using heroin and at the time I was using out in Campbelltown [suburb in South-West Sydney] way, [eventually even] doing it at home with parents and my little sister in the next room.

After discovering drug paraphernalia in the house, Jake's parents removed him from the family home and he moved to the inner city in early 2008: "*I ended up in Kings Cross and with no heroin around or anything and I was staying in a homeless refuge*".

With limited knowledge of the local drug scene, heroin became difficult to acquire and someone he met at the shelter offered him OxyContin®, which Jake had never injected before: "*I didn't know what to do with it so they mixed it up and shot me up*". Jake explains that it was during this time that he developed a great deal of flexibility in his drug consumption. He would use whatever was "*cheaper*" and "*easier to get*". Jake continued to inject an assortment of pharmaceutical and illicit opiates for a majority of the period between 2008 and 2010. During this time, he moved between home detention related to a conviction for a string of burglaries he was involved with, sleeping rough, and a series of unstable housing arrangements. Jake also made several attempts at detoxification and used a range of harm minimization services such as NSP, Sydney's MSIC, and opioid substitution treatment. In late 2010, Jake was stabilized on methadone for a period of approximately two years. He reported first injecting his (prescribed) methadone two months prior to interview, which was followed a week later by a return to intravenous heroin use.

Jake had particular expectations about the ability of a pharmaceutical like OxyContin® to numb his pain, and for a time the medication did fulfill those expectations. He slept better and was able to get on with his life. However, those benefits did not last. After participating in a detoxification program for the first time in 2007, Jake observed a series of shifts in the forms of social support available to him. His friends and family, along with any medical practitioners that found out about his drug use, became constantly skeptical of Jake. He became reluctant to visit the doctor and was eventually asked to leave the family home. These conditions were only exacerbated by difficult feelings of loneliness, for which Jake was using opiates to alleviate.

Once Jake was living on the street, a lack of financial security and uncertain housing arrangements resulted in a form of entrenched loneliness. Jake explains that, during periods of prolonged intravenous use, it is the need to avoid withdrawal that sustains his consumption of opiates:

> I'm just physically addicted to them. Generally don't want to take them and when I do take it I feel like I need to and I don't feel any better until I have taken it. I don't mentally – I don't want it if that makes much sense.

However, Jake goes on to explain that recurring feelings of loneliness often thwart any attempt to remain opiate free:

> But then I detox [and] I'll be fine for a bit, I'll get clean off them again and they send me home and I'm right for a couple of weeks. But like after a while I get lonely and I always go back to them, like I don't know what else to do when I feel like that.

The reliability of the physical sensation that painkillers provide is one way Jake manages the uncertain conditions that characterize cultures of street-based injecting drug use. He explains that: "*if I'm in pain I want to stop it as quickly and easily as possible. That means going and seeing a doctor and getting medication or buying morphine off the street, whatever. I'll do whatever it takes not to be in pain*".

Problematizing Pain

Thus far, this chapter has outlined the lives of three men who have experienced different kinds of pain and had different experiences with painkillers to alleviate that pain. This section will compare the kinds of pain they suffer and the way it has impacted their lives. In summarizing and comparing these men's experiences of pain, this section will also problematize the way physical pain is often separated from emotional pain in general medical discourse and practice.

After a workplace accident in 1999, ongoing physical pain has consistently compromised Allan's capacity to work both in his job and as a volunteer. His condition has also made care for his son more difficult. Alongside the disability of physical pain, Allan explains that the stigma associated with his condition and its treatment is difficult to escape. This stigma has had significant impact on the way Allan himself understands his own medication consumption. Allan is reflective in his observation about the use of analgesics to pre-empt pain, presenting a set of concerns about whether he is using them in the 'wrong way'. Allan elaborates on concerns that he is dependent on pain medications to operate without pain, and that is often a source of stress that can inflame physical pain. This even leads Allan to make tentative comparisons to illicit and addictive consumption.

Mark's descriptions of chronic pain are dominated by the way he subsequently developed an 'addiction' as a result of its treatment. The pain associated with osteomyelitis of the spine made it difficult for Mark to participate in physical labor. In order to keep in work, Mark began to acquire painkillers and eventually heroin from street-based illicit drug markets. More than twenty-five years after his initial hospitalization, Mark now uses painkillers for a complex set of reasons: such as to relieve physical pain and "*make it bearable*"; to stave off withdrawal with a product that is "*guaranteed on the quality*"; to get a euphoric feeling that is "*better than an orgasm*"; and to alleviate the emotional difficulties of "*having to live this illegal sort of underground lifestyle*".

Finally, Jake's example brings into focus a less recognized form of chronic pain. As Jake's story demonstrates, constant emotional suffering can be just as debilitating as persistent physical pain. Indeed, there are many overlaps between Jake's experience of chronic emotional suffering and Allan and Mark's chronic physical pain. Like Allan, pain affected Jake's ability to sleep: painkillers helped Jake forget about Louise's death so that he could ease into sleep. Jake's use of pain medications also affected his life circumstances, eventually informing stigma from family and medical professionals. As was the case for Mark, Jake also felt unable to rely on the medical profession to help him through his pain and subsequent drug dependence. Moreover, Jake's need to avoid the pain of physical withdrawal cannot be separated from the forms of emotional distress that accompany his sense of loss and loneliness.

Mark and Jake's accounts include noteworthy detail about the role of medicine in their dependence on opiates. They describe feeling alienated from treatment services and medical professionals when the issue of substance use became part of how they dealt with the chronic conditions they were experiencing. While Allan's experiences of stigmatization are significant, they do not appear to come directly from medical practitioners and thus seem to have less of an impact on his medical care. This has salient links with sociological observations about the way pain medicine has reformulated addiction in ways that rely on moral assumptions about what pain is and who deserves (opiate) treatment for it. In such accounts, the pain of the 'addict' is constantly delegitimized (Bell and Salmon 2009).

The examples in this chapter demonstrate that people's experience of physical pain, social suffering and emotional anguish can be fluid and interrelated. Chronic pain, whether physical or emotional, is debilitating and thus often means that those who experience it must rely on external structures (such as familial and social support) for their lives to operate smoothly. Medicine is also one of those important structures—providing access to painkillers is the culturally accepted norm for medicine to fulfill its responsibility to alleviate human suffering. However, especially when drug dependence enters the equation, traditional forms of support for those experiencing chronic pain become unreliable and people are often left to fend for themselves—the results can be tragic.

Conclusion

This chapter has explored the way chronic pain and dependence intersect in the lives of three participants. Allan and Mark's examples demonstrate how persistent physical pain can transform people's lives: this involves practical considerations as a result of physical injury, but also the impact of forms of social stigma. Jake's example introduces a less recognized form of chronic emotional pain and highlights the similarities it has with the impacts of physical pain. One of the key elements of the narratives provided by Allan, Mark and Jake is the way chronic pain affects their ability to be productive, or even participate in productive society.

The theme of participation in productive society has noteworthy links to the previous chapter, which focused on the way pain medications are used to increase or sustain productivity at work. Much like the participants in Chapter 5, pleasure also became part of all three men's use of painkillers—albeit to varying degrees. It is important to note that for the participants in this chapter pain relief and pleasure were inseparable experiences: Allan compares the use of pharmaceutical opiates during a flare up of pain to recreational drug use; Mark derives pleasure from release from intense physical and pervasive social stigmatization; Jake began to enjoy the respite from feelings of emotional loss and a deep sense of loneliness when using pain medications. The next chapter engages the notion of 'addiction' more directly by providing a sociological critique of its ability to explain drug use in the lives of two participants. It explores the life histories of two participants who no longer use drugs.

References

Bair, M. J., Wu, J., Damush, T. M., Sutherland, J. M., & Kroenke, K. (2008). Association of Depression and Anxiety Alone and in Combination with Chronic Musculoskeletal Pain in Primary Care Patients. *Psychosomatic Medicine, 70*(8), 890–897.

Bell, K., & Salmon, A. (2009). Pain, Physical Dependence and Pseudoaddiction: Redefining Addiction for 'Nice' People? *International Journal of Drug Policy, 20*(2), 170–178.

Cohen, M., Quintner, J., Buchanan, D., Nielsen, M., & Guy, L. (2011). Stigmatization of Patients with Chronic Pain: The Extinction of Empathy. *Pain Medicine, 12,* 1637–1643.

Collert, S. (1977). Osteomyelitis of the Spine. *Acta Orthopaedica, 48*(3), 283–290.

Crowley-Matoka, M., & True, G. (2012). No One Wants to be the Candy Man: Ambivalent Medicalization and Clinician Subjectivity in Pain Management. *Cultural Anthropology, 27*(4), 689–712.

DePalma, M. J., Ketchum, J. M., & Saullo, T. (2011). What Is the Source of Chronic Low Back Pain and Does Age Play a Role? *Pain Medicine, 12*(2), 224–233.

Dow, C. M., Roche, P. A., & Ziebland, S. (2012). Talk of Frustration in the Narratives of People with Chronic Pain. *Chronic Illness, 8*(3), 176–191.

Fishbain, D. A., Cutler, R., Rosomoff, H. L., & Rosomoff, R. S. (1997). Chronic Pain-Associated Depression: Antecedent or Consequence of Chronic Pain? A Review. *Clinical Journal of Pain, 13*(2), 116–137.

Goffman, E. (1963). *Stigma: Notes on the Management of Spoiled Identity.* Englewood Cliffs, NJ: Prentice-Hall.

Gureje, O., Korff, M. V., Simon, G., & Gater, R. (1998). Persistent Pain and Well-Being: A World Health Organization Study in Primary Care. *Journal of the American Medical Association, 280*(2), 147–152.

Holloway, I., Sofaer-Bennett, B., & Walker, J. (2007). The Stigmatisation of People with Chronic Back Pain. *Disability & Rehabilitation, 29*(18), 1456–1464.

Lupton, D. (2012). *Medicine as Culture: Illness, Disease and the Body.* Thousand Oaks, CA: Sage.

Macrae, W. A. (2001). Chronic Pain After Surgery. *British Journal of Anaesthesia, 87*(1), 88–89.

McCaffery, M., & Thorpe, D. (1989). Differences in Perception of Pain and the Development of Adversarial Relationships among Health Care Providers. In C. S. Hill & W. S. Fields (Eds.), *Advances in Pain Research and Therapy*. New York: Raven.

National Pain Summit Initiative. (2010). *National Pain Strategy: Pain Management for all Australians.* Sydney: MBF Foundation & University of Sydney Pain Management Research Institute.

Reidenberg, M., & Willis, O. (2007). Prosecution of Physicians for Prescribing Opioids to Patients. *Clinical Pharmacology & Therapeutics, 81*(6), 903–906.

Steward, W. T., Herek, G. M., Ramakrishna, J., Bharat, S., Chandy, S., Wrubel, J., et al. (2008). HIV-Related Stigma: Adapting a Theoretical Framework for Use in India. *Social Science & Medicine, 67*(8), 1225–1235.

Thomas, S. P. (2000). A Phenomenologic Study of Chronic Pain. *Western Journal of Nursing Research, 22*(6), 683–705.

Werner, A., & Malterud, K. (2003). It Is Hard Work Behaving as a Credible Patient: Encounters between Women with Chronic Pain and Their Doctors. *Social Science & Medicine, 57*(8), 1409–1419.
Zimmerli, W. (2010). Vertebral Osteomyelitis. *New England Journal of Medicine, 362*(11), 1022–1029.

8

Beyond 'Addiction': Dependence, Injecting and Transitions in Opiate Use

Of the various concerns about non-medical consumption in media and health discourse, dependence on opiates is high on the list. The potential for people who use opiates prescribed by the doctor to become 'hooked' and to subsequently transition to implicitly more 'dangerous' practices such as intravenous or heroin use is a significant theme in health research and media accounts. Such concerns tend to be built on contemporary models of addiction, which assume that prolonged opiate (and other drug) use will result in a linear trajectory of progressive escalation of drug use, as well as associated risk taking and criminal activity. While concern about transition between pharmaceutical and illicit opiates is genuine, it is also often heightened by long-standing and culturally embedded assumptions about who an 'addict' is—typically a male, poor, inner-city urban dweller who uses illicit drugs to satisfy a hedonistic desire for perverse pleasure. Given that opiates can be legitimately prescribed by the doctor and are not always culturally linked to pleasure, this unflattering but culturally entrenched stereotype of who 'the addict' is often fits awkwardly with examples of non-medical consumption. For instance, in an investigative piece on the ABC Four Corners program, reporter Matthew Carney warns that the "misuse of

G. C. Dertadian, *A Fine Line*,
https://doi.org/10.1007/978-981-13-1975-4_8

powerful prescription drugs is creating a new generation of addicts" and a physician interviewed for the program observes that "on the whole, most of these people are indistinguishable - they're not your typical addicts" (2010). The notion that the pharmaceutical opiate addict looks like a 'new' type of addict informs the public attention it receives. Such accounts illustrate the way non-medical use challenges both culturally familiar accounts of addiction, and medical models of dependence.

While concern about dependence may dominate health and media discourse, as we have seen throughout Part II, 'addiction' to pharmaceutical opiates is hardly representative of the way people use painkillers non-medically. For the young people discussed in Chapter 5, painkillers are a consciously chosen alternative to illicit drugs, or are an ideal complement to other forms of recreational drug use. Far from the stereotype of spiraling out of control, these young people carefully and purposefully negotiate the illicit context of their drug use by introducing licit or pharmaceutical substances. Similarly, for participants in Chapter 6, intravenous use and criminal activity do not feature in their experience with non-medical consumption. In fact, the use of painkillers is seen as a way to enhance the legitimate pursuits of productive work and recreational release.

Chapter 7 addressed the issue of drug dependence more directly, focusing on the link between chronic pain and prolonged opiate use. For Allan, Mark and Jake (from the previous chapter), the debilitating effects of chronic pain necessitate their continued use of opiate medications. This also has important links to the historical and conceptual developments of addiction discussed in Part I. The study of addiction incorporates moralizing distinctions based on structural factors such as race and class. For instance, middle-class housewives and doctors during the middle of last century in North America were thought of as 'normal people' who had become addicted 'accidently' through medical treatment (Acker 2002). By contrast, impoverished young black men were regarded as 'psychopaths' whose addiction was the result of 'hedonism'. Throughout the remainder of the century, these moral distinctions were formalized in medical models of addiction through an emphasis on the physiological and psychological elements of the emerging 'brain disease model' of addiction.

This chapter addresses the limitations of addiction as a framework for understanding the use of opiates by drawing on the life histories of two participants who no longer use drugs. The chapter begins by reviewing sociological accounts of addiction that highlight conceptual critiques of medical models of addiction. It then details the life history of a participant named 'Emma' to illustrate general critiques of addiction provided by the sociological literature. The chapter then moves on to critically assess the issue of transition (between opiates and modes of administration) in the epidemiological literature regarding non-medical pharmaceutical opiate use. Following this, the story of a participant called 'Felix' is introduced to illustrate the limitations of the notion of transition. Finally, the chapter addresses the idea of 'loss of control' by critically discussing agency in injecting drug use as a key element of thinking beyond the framework of addiction.

The Sociology of Addiction

Until recently the social sciences had been reluctant to engage with the concept of 'addiction'. Two central concerns underpin sociology's lack of interest in addiction: the first is the way addiction is embedded in therapeutic frameworks that belie the sociological tendency to problematize the medical designation of social problems (Weinberg 2011); the second is to avoid reproducing the moralizing discourses that characterize 'out of control' consumption as a betrayal of the modernist value of restraint (Lenson 1999). These are significant critiques that need to be taken seriously in any sociological engagement with addiction. However, even given such hesitations many sociologists have come to recognize that empirical evidence does suggest that a small minority of people who use drugs describe and demonstrate a sense of 'loss of control' and that this cannot simply be explained as being imposed by agents of social control. This section will canvas a set of literature that has come to be termed the sociology of addiction.

Despite being somewhat less developed than the sociological literature on drug use and drug cultures, there have been important sociological studies that have directly addressed addiction. One of the first, and certainly the most influential sociological study of addiction was Alfred Lindesmith's (1938) study of heroin users. Based on interviews with approximately fifty "heroin addicts", Lindesmith developed a theoretical account of addiction, arguing that a conscious recognition of the use of opiates to stave off withdrawal defined the 'addict':

> Any satisfactory theory must attempt to account for the fact that the repeated administration of opiates sometimes is followed by addiction and sometimes is not. The factor which accounts for this differential effect appears to be the person's knowledge or belief, supplied him [sic] by his cultural milieu, concerning the nature of the distress that accompanies the sudden cessation of the opiate. If he fails to realize the connection between this distress and the opiate he escapes addiction, whereas if he attributes the discomfort to the opiate and thereafter uses the opiate to alleviate it he invariably becomes addicted. (1938: 593)

For Lindensmith, addiction was a social process by which people who use drugs only became an 'addict' when reflecting back the cultural stereotype by consciously using opiates to 'stave off withdrawal'.

Lindesmith's most significant contribution is found in the way this seminal study (and subsequent work) demonstrated that people have meaningful responses to drug use that cannot be reduced to the pharmacological effects of drugs on the body (Maher and Dertadian 2018). A range of functionalist contributions during the 1960s extended Lindesmith's theory by describing addiction as a rationally calculated response to socio-structural disadvantage (Ray 1961; Cloward and Ohlin 1960). These kinds of functionalist accounts tended, however, to be largely conservative and thus conceived of addiction as a deviance that required 'correction' (Weinberg 2011: 301).

As part of a broader rejection of functionalist sociology during the second half of the twentieth century, qualitative traditions of the sociology of deviance entered, what Matza (1969) calls an 'appreciative' turn in drug research. Qualitative drugs research from the 1960s onward has attempted to empathize with those labeled 'deviants' and especially 'addicts'. During the height of its influence in the 1970s, the labeling perspective in sociology and criminology tended to present addiction as an internalized identity imposed by agents of social control. Sociologists of deviance thus often engaged people who describe themselves as 'addicts', yet only ever addressed addiction in ambiguous ways that reduced it to a label.

Denzin (1987) was one of the only labeling theorists to treat addiction as worthy of genuine sociological study. In his work on alcoholism, the 'emotionally divided self' played a key role in his theorization of addiction. Denzin contends that alcoholics are internally conflicted about their consumption of alcohol and that this internal conflict is reflective of broader social conditions that both encourage its consumption and reject its overconsumption. In this account, compulsive alcohol use is presented as part of a social context that produces the particular conditions under which 'addiction' to alcohol emerges.

Social constructionist perspectives have also extended Denzin's theorization of addiction by arguing that the practices that make up 'addiction' are necessarily embedded in the conditions of late-modernity. That is to say, not only does 'addiction' have social determinants but it is 'unintelligible outside the nexus of cultural practices and beliefs within which it is found' (Weinberg 2011: 304). For instance, Levine (1978) argued that the Temperance movements of the early twentieth century produced demands about self-control and an accountability to economic responsibility, for which the pathology of 'alcoholism' emerged as an answer. Acker (2002) argues that a series of social and political movements in North America collectively constituted "the classical era of narcotic control", which subsequently produces the concept of and the practices that comprise the urban 'junkie'.

The work of Keane also makes important contributions to the social constructionist perspective through a poststructuralist analysis of discourse, and its role in assembling the various elements of addiction discourse into a stable biomedical entity. Keane's analysis of addiction discourse has highlighted its expansion to other forms of strong attachments and habitual practices that are not limited to drug use (such as gambling, exercise, sex, food, etc.) (Fraser et al. 2014; Keane 2002). This can be partly explained by changes to the way 'addiction' is formulated in contemporary medicine, with medical discourse constantly expanding the reach of what is 'addictive' and what it means to be 'addicted'. This has also contributed to, what Sedgwick (1993) refers to as an epidemic of "addiction attribution", in which there has been a proliferation of human behaviors deemed to be addictive: some recent examples include "'workaholism', 'shopaholism', 'being sexual compulsive', 'relationship addiction', 'exercise addiction', and the all too self-aware 'self-help addiction'" (O'Toole and Connect 2013: 25).

A sociological approach to addiction requires a problematization of medical accounts of addiction that present it to be a stable or fixed disease state. The sociological perspective thus complicates the linear narrative of transition from 'normal' to 'pathological', focusing instead on the structures that produce and the discourses that define or reinforce compulsive/dependent consumption. The next section will provide an example of a young woman whose history with drug use confirms elements of the medical model of addiction, but also illustrates how this model hinges upon structural factors and discursive constructions that do not always hold true. While 'Emma's example should not be thought of as representative of the experience of people who become drug dependent, her stories do highlight some of the key limitations of the framework of addiction outlined in this section.

Emma: "I Never Did Any of That Stuff"

Emma grew up in a wealthy suburb on Sydney's affluent Lower North Shore. Still in her early twenties, the usually smooth road from a seemingly privileged adolescence to a university-educated young adulthood was filled with difficult and unexpected circumstances. Her drug use commenced with smoking cannabis at 14 for "*calming down [and] chilling out*". She also took Xanax® from her parent's bathroom cabinet and snorted them to "*kill anxiety*" and "*just as like jokes or whatever on the weekend*". By the age of 16, Emma was also regularly mixing alcohol and Panadeine Forte®.

It was at this time that she met a charismatic young man named 'Tom', who was only one year her senior. A year into their relationship, Tom sustained a debilitating back injury for which he was prescribed

Panadeine Forte® and OxyContin®. After months without relief Tom started to become depressed, in part because of his incapacitation from the injury, and the pair began crushing and snorting his prescriptions: "*my whole using [history], I had my partner, so you'll hear me refer to him a lot*". After a few months, Emma and Tom were regularly snorting pharmaceutical opiates like OxyContin® and MS-Contin®, which they continued to acquire from a friend who worked at a pharmacy. In the midst of a fierce divorce at the time, both of Tom's parents kicked him out of their respective homes. As he moved in with Emma, the pair continued to escalate their use of prescription opiates: "*[it] would be more to yeah just get high and relax… We'd just eat them [OxyContin®] and watch a movie and ate pizza*".

The next year of Emma's life involved a noticeable shift in her relationship with Tom and the medications they had been consuming together. As Tom's injury worsened, his depression deepened and he started to become abusive toward Emma: "*not abuse as in violent abuse, but he became very abusive… I mean you would rather be punched in the face than have these things said to you*". After a little under a year of oral and intranasal opiate use the couple's tolerance had grown significantly and Tom insisted that they start injecting the pharmaceuticals: "*by the end of it we would never swallow the pills, we would always crush them, taking the binders off, and shooting [injecting] them*". Though the couple had been dysfunctional for many months, the move to intravenous use put a serious strain on Emma and Tom's relationship.

Over the next six months, Tom's abuse became more frequent and more extreme. He began to demand that Emma go out and buy drugs for him:

> It would always be "I don't wonna leave" and he'd get really depressed and so he didn't want to leave the house. And so I always had to do it by myself, I always had to go to the city and everything. And I'm a pretty small girl, I'm 5 foot. It's not too hard to go "yeah I'm gonna pick you up and steal you".

Emma was 17 at the time. After a period of approximately 8 months of injecting OxyContin® and MS-Contin®, in August of 2008, one of the several "*dealers*" that Emma bought drugs from was not able to supply any oxycodone product and suggested she buy some heroin instead: "*when we ran out of the pharmaceuticals and stuff we moved on to heavy drugs, so we moved on to the gear and the heroin and whatever*".

After several months of intravenous heroin use, Emma's family began placing increasing pressure on her to leave Tom. Her growing resentment over Tom's abuse and demands eventually culminated in a dramatic end to their relationship. Emma asked Tom to leave the family home and cut ties with him, before entering a rehabilitation facility for opiate dependence. At the time of interview, Emma had not used any opiate for a period of 18 months. She is currently studying an undergraduate degree at university.

On reflecting about her time injecting opiates, Emma places distance between her own experience injecting drugs and those of 'other' people, who were "*your typical kind of junkie*". She goes on to explain that "*normally [when I] tell people that I had a problem with heroin they go 'Pffft yeah ok'. And they even did when I was using*". Emma also speaks about never becoming homeless, never participating in sex work, never having to steal and never being convicted of any crime throughout her time using opiates:

> I wouldn't be able to name any other female in the room [at rehab] who hasn't at some stage had sex with somebody for money or drugs, hasn't robbed someone, hasn't done all this stuff. [Other participants in the rehabilitation program] are like "yeah, yeah you must of done this or that"… No, no. I just dealt pot and worked 20 plus a week.

Emma is adamant in insisting that her experiences injecting drugs do not fulfill the stereotype. For instance, when talking about Tom, she recalls: "*He stole from the family, which I just think is wrong anyway. I wouldn't steal from my Mum. He is the stereotype sociopath… I never did any of that stuff. I would never*".

Emma's trajectory of opiate use is structured in many ways by her middle-class status. She explains:

> In the Lower North Shore everyone's parents have it in their cupboard. I probably wouldn't be able to name one of my friend's parent's who isn't on Xanax, or Valium, or at least have it just in case.

The 'legitimate' prescription of opiates and other pharmaceuticals is widespread in affluent suburbs of Sydney. These medications are used to deal with a range of emotional problems and social difficulties, and, as Emma described, most often seem to be used preventatively. The omnipresence of pharmaceuticals in the middle-class homes that Emma grew up surrounded by thus inform a partial legitimization of the use of pain medications for emotional suffering: "*So I guess for me using numbed the pain or prevented it*".

Emma's experience with opiates also has clearly gendered elements. She describes a concerted effort to avoid any visible sign of her drug use, and thus, the impression that she is a 'classless' or 'improper' woman. When comparing herself to "*more serious*" drug users and other women who use heroin, Emma says that "*I used to be a bit more delicate and careful*". She made sure to inject in places that could be easily concealed and always used clean injecting equipment. She also discusses how Tom's abusive behavior mitigates the responsibility she bares for her drug use:

> It's hard because I believe in the concept of not 100% blame. So in these statements, I say that 'yes, it was my fault'. But I was in a really abusive relationship, and it was painful, it was really painful.

Emma's account of being drawn into increasingly intense drug use through a relationship with a charismatic and controlling man only partly conforms to dominant discourses of women as vulnerable victims of both sexuality and drugs (Campbell and Ettorre 2011). Emma insists that she made her own choices about drug use, but that those choices were made in concert with the circumstances of her relationship. This is not to deny the impact of abusive intimate relationships in women's lives and the connections between abuse, violence and drug use (Wingood et al. 2000), but rather to further contextualize the way agency of women is experienced.

It is also worth noting that Emma's class position intersects with her gender in ways that made the exercise of agency within the relationship possible. She was not economically dependent on Tom. The structures of her upbringing and the support of her family allowed her to exit the relationship with relative ease. She also had immediate access to a quality rehabilitation program, with the support of her family: "*I was really lucky, I mean I was in rehab with people coming down off OxyContin® and stuff, and Jesus Christ! They did it so tough. I was really lucky*". As a result, Emma is able conceptualize her drug use as confined to a discrete but difficult period of her life, which she has now firmly put behind her: "*So I had a problem and I went to a rehab for that and umm… and I guess that was like two years ago. And now I'm working and I go to Uni*".

From Pharmaceutical Opiates to Heroin

In the epidemiological literature, non-medical use of pharmaceutical opiates in the US in particular paints a picture that is unfamiliar to most health and drug researchers. Opiate overdose trends in the US have seen the largest increases in deaths among populations that have had traditionally low rates of drug use; including Caucasians, the middle-aged, those in the middle class and women (Rudd et al. 2016; Bohnert et al. 2011). The US context has also seen significant increases in emergency room presentations related to opiate overdose (Yokell et al. 2014) and opiate dependence treatment (Carise et al. 2007) among these populations. This has raised concern among health practitioners that non-medical use of and dependence on pharmaceutical medications may be changing the face of drug addiction and thus the way we can respond to it. Part of the concern about these 'non-traditional' drug users lies with the possibility that people who are dependent on pharmaceutical opiates may also use or transitions to illicit opiates such as heroin. This section will canvas epidemiological literature about transitions between licit and illicit opiates and provide a critique of its limitations.

As discussed earlier, one of the central components of mainstream addiction discourse as well as a prominent feature of biomedical accounts of addiction has been the notion of transition—from 'normal' person to 'addict', from a 'healthy' to an 'addicted' brain. The introduction of this chapter touched on some of the media rhetoric about the apparent threat of OxyContin® (and other pharmaceuticals) transforming otherwise 'normal' people into desperate 'drug addicts'. Part I of the book outlined how medical models of addiction claim that the use of drugs (like OxyContin® and heroin) alters the neurochemistry of the brain to create a 'pathological' desire for the pleasures of drug use. This notion of ontological or biochemical transition to addiction also informs epidemiological research about transitions from licit to illicit opiates. Here it is worth recalling the historical and social construction of distinctions between licit and illicit opiates. There is no necessary pharmacological distinction between OxyContin® and heroin that makes dependence to the latter more likely. There are, however, important considerations to be made about involvement in the political economy of the illicit drug market and criminalized cultures of injecting drug use. While the epidemiological literature ostensibly uses the term 'transition' in a neutral way, to simply indicate movement from one drug to another, a moralizing ontological politics pervades this literature's concern with the distinction between licit and illicit opiate consumption.

While qualitative literature about processes of transition in the Australian context is limited (Dertadian and Maher 2013), an emerging set of North American studies have begun to document transitions from the non-medical or recreational use of pharmaceutical opiates to intravenous and heroin use. This literature tends to present the non-medical use of pharmaceutical opiates as a serious public health problem (and even as an 'epidemic'), in part by describing a link between the increased availability and non-medical use of opiate medications with increases in injecting drug use and heroin use (Compton et al. 2016; Kolodny et al. 2015). For instance, in one study 39% of young heroin users reported being "hooked on" prescription opiates before using heroin (Peavy et al. 2012). Another study, which reported a similar rate of non-medical pharmaceutical opiate use prior to heroin use, found that most who reported this were also less likely to be familiar with safe injecting and drug treatment services, as well as being less likely to be tested for infectious diseases (Pollini et al. 2011). This is complimented by research which also indicates that many of the country's youngest generation of heroin users were first introduced to opiates through pharmaceuticals (Carlson et al. 2016; McCabe et al. 2007).

The theme of escalation in studies that trace a path from pharmaceutical opiates to heroin readily feeds into a medical model of addiction, in which dependence necessarily drives more harmful and deviant practices, until the user loses control of both their consumption and their lives in general. These studies draw on classic accounts of the disease model of the heroin user continually returning to the drug to stave off withdrawal, but simply add a new pre-heroin 'gateway' element. A 2007 study from the US directly poses the question: "Is OxyContin® a "Gateway Drug"?" The study found that OxyContin® itself is unlikely to cause escalating drug consumption, but that poly-opiate use, as well as poly-drug use more generally, is associated with quicker progression to intravenous and heroin consumption (Grau et al. 2007). While evidence of a plausible causal link is sparse, it is clear that current data does suggest that, among a minority in the US, the non-medical use of pharmaceutical opiates may represent a 'new' pathway to heroin and injecting drug use (Degenhardt et al. 2010).

In a recent qualitative study of people who inject drugs in Montreal, the authors observed that the proportion of participants reporting the injection of pharmaceutical opiates increased from 21% to 75% between 2005 and 2009, while the prevalence of other drugs like heroin and crack use remained stable (Bruneau et al. 2012). Similarly, in a study of pharmaceutical opiate use among street-based young injecting drug users (aged 16–25 years) in Los Angeles and New York City, Lankenau and colleagues found that 82% of respondents had first used pharmaceutical opiates non-medically through oral ingestion prior to injecting (Lankenau et al. 2012). Just over 80% of the sample of this study also reported non-medical pharmaceutical opiate use prior to first injecting heroin. Beyond rates of use, qualitative studies also provide more detail about the nature and meaning of these transitions. In another qualitative study about opiate transition, users express dismay and surprise at each stage of progression from seemingly unproblematic pill use to more taboo and risker forms of drug use (Mars et al. 2014). The authors describe this less as movement through gateways, and more as a process involving 'the crossing of thresholds of stigmatized behavior'—from crushing to sniffing pills, from smoking to injecting heroin (2014: 261). These data also suggest that although most non-medical pharmaceutical opiate consumption often begins with oral ingestion, a minority in the US may transition to the administration of opiates by injection and/or the use of heroin, typically within 2–3 years of initial use (Lankenau et al. 2012).

Though the issue of opiate transition represents a genuine concern for public health, it is also important to contextualize the cultural specificity of this phenomena in the US. In 1996, Purdue Pharma released and began aggressively marketing its new extended release opiate product OxyContin® in the US (Berge and Burkle 2014). At the same time, the Pharmaceutical Industry also lobbied for the introduction of mandatory pain assessment (Meldrum 2016), facilitating a more liberal prescribing environment for pharmaceutical opiates (Schofferman et al. 2014). This resulted in the increased availability of pharmaceutical opiates, which also began to be used non-medically (Johnson and Schardan 2012). These conditions produced the circumstances under which significant increases in overdose related to opiates sparked public health officials to declare an 'opioid epidemic', as well as a series of regulator measures to reduce the availability and ability to 'abuse'pharmaceutical opiates. This includes the introduction of 'tamper-resistant' formulations of opiate medications (Chilcoat et al. 2014; Vosburg et al. 2013), the establishment of real-time monitoring of pharmaceutical purchases and crackdowns on illicit 'pill mills' operations (Kuehn 2014). While such measures may have been well intentioned, there is also evidence to suggest that the sudden reduced availability of pharmaceutical opiates may have encouraged transitions to heroin use (Dart et al. 2015; Mars et al. 2014; Cicero et al. 2012). Thus, the picture painted by epidemiological research in the US about opiate transition is informed by the specific history of how opiates became widely available and then suddenly scarcely available. This has not been the case in Australia.

In the Australian context, pharmaceutical analgesics have not been the subject of comparably aggressive marketing and lobbying efforts, which has meant that less young people have been prescribed or had to access pharmaceutical opiates for non-medical use (Nicholas et al. 2011). While Australia has seen exponential increases in opiate prescribing in the period between 1992 and 2012 (Blanch et al. 2014), this did not translate into significant increases in rates of overdose from prescribed opiates, especially when compared to heroin (Roxburgh et al. 2011). However, since 2008 there has been a steady increase in overdose deaths related to pharmaceutical opiates, largely driven by increases in Fentanyl overdose (Roxburgh et al. 2017). Australian data also indicate that people who inject pharmaceutical opiates tend to have an established history of heroin use before initiating pharmaceutical opiate injecting (Nielsen et al. 2015; Degenhardt et al. 2006). This is not of course to suggest that transitions between licit and illicit opiates do not occur, but that a more complex understandings of such transitions is required.

Indeed, there are aspects of the case studies cover in this and the previous chapter that are worth revisiting for the qualitative detail they add. There are aspects of Emma's experience with opiates that can provide important complements to current epidemiological data about transitions between opiates. Emma's transition between opiates was a largely linear process, from OxyContin® to intravenous then heroin use, before entering rehabilitation and abstaining from opiate use for 18 months at the time of interview. However, it is important to consider how this linear transition may be structured by Emma's middle-class status. The availability of pharmaceutical opiates in her own home and the homes of friends means that pharmaceutical medications can be thought of as 'soft' or 'safe' drugs. This reinforces the notion that heroin is a 'hard' or 'dangerous' drug that is unfamiliar and thus threatening to the middle-class milieu of Sydney's North Shore. This certainly had an impact on the way Emma related to addiction. For Emma, she never became a 'proper' addict, because that would have involved sex work, theft and deceit of her family—these were the practices of a different group of people that "*totally fulfilled the stereotype*".

In considering the classed elements of Emma's experience, it is also worth comparing them to that of other participants who transitioned from or between pharmaceutical opiates and heroin. Mark and Jake, introduced in the previous chapter, both began by using pharmaceutical opiates for pain and transitioned to intravenous and heroin use. Mark's continued use of pharmaceutical opiates outside the prescriptions of his physicians related mainly to the need to work, as well as the physical nature of his work. Similarly, his transitions to intravenous and heroin use are marked by the bodily demands of physical labor, which Mark explains is "*the only thing I know how to do*". Mark's attempts at detoxification and rehabilitation were many, but were largely unsuccessful. That he has a strained relationship with his family and says "*I have no meaningful relationship with anyone anymore*", is telling of the lack of emotional support he would have been able to drawn upon in attempts to reduce his drug use.

Unlike Emma, Jake's drug use does not occur in clearly identifiable stages that can be neatly described as discrete transitions from oral to intravenous pharmaceutical opiates use and to heroin injection. Jake began using pharmaceutical opiates orally for approximately 18 months before entering a detoxification program. This was followed by a single instance of intravenous methadone use, then with periodic heroin injection. Following 6 months of house arrest, where Jake did not use opiates, he began injecting OxyContin® while living in a homeless refuge. For years after being forced to leave his family home in a disadvantaged suburb of Sydney's South-West, Jake injected heroin and a wide range of pharmaceutical opiates interchangeably based on "*what ever is available and good at the time*". Following a period of stabilization on methadone, Jake gave into a deep sense of loneliness and injected his prescribed dose, which was followed by a further period of intravenous heroin use. For Jake, attempts at sobriety have been multiple and their success is described as partial and semi-permanent.

Support from family and friends, stable housing arrangements, as well as physical and conceptual distance from the criminalized/stigmatized context of street-based injecting drug use are all components of Emma's life that are not available to Mark and Jake.

Such comparisons demonstrate that epidemiological literature may benefit from complementary qualitative assessments of the complex life events and life circumstances that inform people's use of opiates. Qualitative data do not only provide complimentary insight into the complex individual circumstances and significant structural determinants of the trajectory of a person's opiate use, it can also provide alternative accounts that do not fit the narratives of linear transition, from pharmaceutical opiate to injecting and then heroin use. As the next case study demonstrates, people can have a very different experience of transition to those included in the epidemiological literature canvassed here.

Felix: "You Don't Know Where the Line Is Until You've Crossed It"

At the time of interview Felix was 31 years old. The first thing Felix shared in the interview was an explanation that, for many years before using pharmaceutical opiates he regularly injected heroin. He spoke in short considered bursts with a calm tone of voice that seemed to mask the chaos that had characterized significant parts of his adult life. Felix had spent years in and out of the medical and social services that are scattered around the inner-city of Sydney and in counseling with mental health professionals. From the outset, it was clear that Felix had engaged in an intense inner dialogue, over many years, about his own life choices. His considered responses left the lasting impression that, had he been born to a different life, Felix would have taken to intellectual pursuits with great ease. However, the circumstances of Felix's life meant that he identified as an 'addict': "*I always conscientiously tried to stay out of the drug scene, but I was an addict so I don't know where that leaves you*".

Felix spent most of his adult life living in the heart of Sydney's infamous Kings Cross region. Having spent so much time there Felix developed a foundation of friendships and relationships that characterized his late-teens and most of his twenties. Felix first injected heroin at the age of 19. His friends from the area made up a large part of that journey: "*it started off with interesting people, good friends of mine, intelligent kids, musicians you know*". Felix also started dating a young woman named Lisa around this time, who he met as part of this circle of friends. Though he had injected heroin prior to dating Lisa, it was his time using with her that made drug use a 'normal' part of Felix's life: "*she made everything speed up and got me in a lot deeper a lot quicker than I would've normally I think... It all just became normal when I was with Lisa*".

Felix described Lisa as a "*thrill seeker*" with a "*troubled past*". She was popular among his friends, and Felix felt a kind of privilege that she would choose him as her partner. Lisa acted as a kind of benchmark for the group: "*I always knew she was way further down the road than me, but while ever she was ok and trying to struggle [through], it felt like we were all kind of protected*". As the pair became more and more immersed in the drug scene, Felix's father rapidly pulled him out in May of 2003. Felix was put on a plane to Israel, where he was forced to sober up without any form of detoxification: "*he just sent me off to Israel. So I got on a plane and went to Israel and just didn't sleep for a week*".

On his return from Israel Felix and Lisa started to drift apart, and as a result he delved deeper into the drug use. His use of heroin soon became a lifestyle. Felix suffered through a tumultuous few years moving between homelessness and crisis accommodation for the period between 2004 and 2009. He survived this period of intense drug and lifestyle change by engaging in harm minimization peer education and utilizing a range of drug treatment programs. However, this period of Felix's life had a lasting impact on his sense of self-worth. When describing unsatisfactory encounters with counselors Felix reflects:

> I've had people tell me before "oh you're so complex and intelligent" and this and that. That doesn't really help you at all. That really messes with your head if anything. I mean thinking that you're smart doesn't do you any favors.

Felix felt that his decision to inject heroin excluded him from the realm of intelligent, productive society and that a journey toward sobriety was the only path to that goal.

In 2009, Felix decided to switch from heroin to injecting pharmaceutical opiates as part of an attempt to regulate his opiate intake more easily. Felix reflects:

> I was using them for a long time, OxyContin® and MS-Contin® I mean, as a replacement originally for heroin". Felix recalled that being able to know how the drug was made and what dose he was injecting meant "it felt safer".

He goes to on to say that "*heroin quality fluctuated so much it was so hard to work out what you're getting… So OxyContin® became a far more stable thing for most of the Cross*". Establishing a more regulated relationship with his opiate intake was significant for Felix:

> Once you're addicted you need the stuff to function, so you know you're in no position to ask hospitals for it or anything but you generally do need some kind of opiate or synthetic opiate to function. But if you don't [know] what you're getting then it's hard to manage it… Oxys give you that certainty.

His transition to pharmaceutical opiate injecting was also accompanied by taking up a range of other harm minimization services. Felix started visiting Sydney's MSIC more often and he began administering his pharmaceutical opiates with a 'cold wash' method recommended by the staff there: "*[you] do a cold wash up at the Injecting Centre because it's healthier*".

Indeed, Felix reveals how he owes his life to the culture of harm minimization that has come to characterize much of the health and social services of Sydney's Kings Cross district: "*those services are good because it makes you feel like you can help people and yourself, like you forgot you're even capable of that*". Yet in trying to come to terms with the moral weight attached to his time injecting drugs on the street, Felix also comments that: "*I was involved in a lot of… harm minimization and peer to peer education. So the line gets really blurry between that and the fact that everything that you're doing is illegal*". Felix describes an internal conflict about how to reconcile the illegality of his drug use alongside, what he regards to be, the necessity of peer education of harm minimization. This internal conflict is reflective of broader debates about the role of harm minimization and its potential to apparently encourage 'risky' drug-taking practices.

After approximately 8 months injecting pharmaceutical opiates Felix enrolled in a methadone program and began looking for work. Having learnt how to manage his own opiate intake with pharmaceutical opiates was described as an important part of his success in the methadone program. In describing the six months before he was stabilized on methadone Felix remarked: "*ultimately I'd be looking for [OxyContin®] to keep myself together so I could function*". As he began to seriously consider a life without drugs, Felix reflected:

> You get this horrible tiny little window where you can function. But then if you're too stoned obviously at job interviews and things you look terrible. Whereas if you don't have anything that day you're sick and then you're not able to do anything. So you've got this horrible little window that you can function.

His use of painkillers was thus an important way in which he could gain some level of control over the window of functionality.

The way Felix was using pharmaceutical opiates has clear links to the way methadone is prescribed to people who are dependent on opiates. Felix's use of pharmaceutical opiates can be thought of as part of a personalized form of opiate maintenance. Indeed, after entering a methadone program in 2010, Felix made comparisons to his use of painkillers and the treatment he was undertaking:

> while [methadone] stabilizes the use of these things it's still – I'm on that side of the opiate divide… Like there's this whole process of getting sick and detox that I can't go through. In some ways its pretty similar to the way I was using the Oxys, except it's not illegal now.

Felix was stabilized on methadone for 18 months before transitioning off the medication to become opiate free:

> I got a really good doctor that took me on… I was lucky enough to get on the program and then lucky enough that my doctor, when he moved out – because he'd had enough of doing outreach – so he took me across to his practice and so I'm just one of his actual patients now.

His use of painkillers is in part a response to the precariousness of the medical and health services available to those who are drug dependent. The injecting of pharmaceutical opiates was an improvised appropriation of the kind of medical maintenance (methadone) programs that are not easy to get access to, and for which it is difficult to find "*a good doctor who actually gives a fuck*".

Felix's example is illustrative of how the surveillance and policing of people who inject drugs is often prioritized over a minimization of the harms of drug use (Keane 2003). For Felix, practices of improvised self-care (through injecting opiates as replacement therapy) and care for others (through peer-to-peer education) emerge as important ways to maintain health and social support. These practices of care are not, however, ideal, and Felix's account of them is not romanticized. He spoke about difficultly reconciling the difference between his use for anxiety, pleasure and to regulate dependence:

> I started feeling a lot of anxiety, and the withdrawals just make that worse. So originally it seemed to make a relief from that which was great… But like I said that line between just use and dependency is really hard to work out. You don't know where the line is until you've crossed it.

In saying so, there are a series of significant personal and social meanings that are associated with Felix's use of painkillers that cannot be explained by a language of 'abuse' nor the concept of addiction. Where the medical/epidemiological literature prioritizes the avoidance of any intravenous drug use, and its associated harms, people who inject drugs are more likely to worry about how to avoid arrest or overdose.

The significance of qualitative assessment is highlighted by Felix's encounters with pharmaceutical opiate injection. Survey data and other epidemiological research about transition are unlikely to capture alternative reasons for why people inject these medications outside of a general 'pathway' to 'heroin addiction'. For Felix, pharmaceutical opiate injection was a way to stabilize his use of opioids, on his own terms. The use of pharmaceutical injection set him up well to manage methadone treatment and eventually stop using opiates altogether. Felix's example thus raises complex questions about the different stages of his use and how addiction factors into them. Does his use of pharmaceutical opiates to regulate opiate intake represent a continuation or disruption of his addiction? What then does this mean for his use of methadone for 18 months? How are we to understand his subsequent detoxification and sobriety? Is it possible that Felix injected painkillers to 'get clean'?

Agency in Injecting Drug Use

A central theme of addiction discourse and the way it is applied to the notion of transition between licit and illicit opiates is the notion of control. How much control do people who use drugs have? What does drug use do to one's ability to control the amount and type of opiate use? The notion of 'loss of control' has long been central to addiction discourse for some time (Foddy and Savulescu 2010). Definitions of addiction and clinical diagnosis relating to substance use have often centered on the idea that the 'addict' is 'out of control'. The most recent version of the DSM includes diagnostic criteria directly related to 'control'. 'Impaired control' refers to the patient's inability to self-determine the amount of drug consumed. 'Social impairment' relates to the patient's inability to manage drug use to the detriment of work or other social activities. 'Risky use' indicates that the patient is unable to avoid drug-taking practices detrimental to their health. Biomedical models of addiction as 'brain disease' also indicate that prolonged drug use impairs the brain's ability to make decisions about present and future drug consumption.

Despite a medical focus on 'lack of control' much public health policy and harm minimization advocacy has focused on empowering people who inject drugs to make healthier choices about their drug consumption. Sometimes this comes in the form of hard fought battle to provide social services to support people who inject drugs, while other times it involves a more moralistic rhetorical deferral to the individual to 'take responsibility' for apparently autonomous choices about drug use. This section develops a conceptual discussion of the agentive capacity of people who inject drugs, as a way of exploring the tension between structure and agency found in medical discourse and public policy, as well as the lives of Emma and Felix. At the outset, it is key to note that neoliberal discourse also utilizes an emphasis on individual responsibility for health. As noted in Chapter 2, a defining moment for the harm minimization movement was the establishment of needle and syringe programs in the UK. The Thatcher government's neoliberal policy agenda, which sought to make people who inject drugs responsible for their own health, provided a political framework that allowed access to sterile-injecting equipment. While harm minimization has evolved into a broader social movement quite distinct from neoliberalism, the ability to empower the individual remains an important feature.

A set of critical literatures has since sought to engage and problematize neoliberal discourse in health promotion about harm minimization. Neoliberal health promotion often places a discursive focus on empowering people who inject drugs. Some scholars have actively embraced neoliberalism in order to position injecting drug users within broader frameworks of legitimate consumption. FitzGerald and colleagues have, for instance, argued that a neoliberal reframing of people who use drugs allows for the ability to install them with 'all the characteristics of non-drug users, the only different being that they consume an illegal commodity' (1999: 2). Of course the consumption of an illegal commodity, or the consumption of a licit commodity under illicit contexts, has important consequences that cannot be overlooked. In Moore's study of public health material related to overdose prevention, he notes that people who inject drugs are presented as 'individualized, rational, autonomous agent[s]… "free" to choose to change 'risky' injecting practices' (2004: 1554). He goes on to suggest that this emphasis on the individual capacity to 'choose' not to engage in 'risky' injecting practices is at odds with ethnographic evidence that, within the "cultural logics of street-based IDUs [injecting drug users], there are many valid reasons for continuing to engage in practices that put them at risk of heroin overdose and other drug-related harm" (2004: 1554).

Fraser and Seear's work on hepatitis C and its transmission among people who inject drugs has noted that public health literature assumes that the "individual can and must control their health and that reducing incidence is primarily an individual responsibility" (2013: 4). The authors argue that the individual is central to contemporary public health, especially as it relates to hepatitis C and injecting drug use. However, the individual is more than simply a rhetorical device in health promotion. The notion of the self-determining responsible individual is also a tool of governance that is both deployed by state authorities that seek to govern at a distance, and internalized by subjects. Fraser notes elsewhere that "the primacy of the individual in western culture is indeed reflected in hepatitis C and safe injecting materials, and... for a range of reasons, injecting drug users also make use of notions of individual responsibility" (2004: 200).

The assumed capacity to make 'healthy' choices is thus at odds with much of the medical literature's emphasis on the way drug use impairs the agentive capacity of people who are drug dependent. This is particularly problematic when considering that much public health literature claims to be informed by the most current developments in addiction science and medicine. Moreover, the focus on individual responsibility in much public health literature ignores an abundance of qualitative research that suggests that the agentive capacity of people who inject drugs, for instance, is often mitigated by important socio-structural barriers. Fraser (2008) and Moore's (2004) work has often advocated for a cautious negotiation of the messages of empowerment that make services like needle and syringe programs possible, as well as a recognition of the social structures that mediate the individual's access to such resources. They recommend:

> mobilisation of the neo-liberal subject in relation to drug users, producing analysis that acknowledges the value of doing so, but calling for the need to consider the context in which the subject operates in conceptualising the responsibilities and capacities of the individual drug user. (Moore and Fraser 2006: 3040)

Keane's (2003) critique of the harm minimization philosophy provides a slightly different approach that does not rely on an oscillation between the denial or empowerment of agency. For Keane, the 'freedom' of people who use drugs is not a preexisting state that can simply be allowed or denied by public health policy. Instead, Keane argues that agency is a socially constituted capacity produced and mediated by an assortment of discourses, policies and personal circumstances. Keane's approach provides a compelling framework for explaining the agentive capacity of people who inject drugs, especially as it relates to the lives of Emma and Felix.

In interviews with people who inject drugs in this study, a sense of self-sufficiency was often foregrounded. Marginalization from traditional forms of social and medical support produces an intense reliance on the individual. Emma is adamant in her insistence that, even during her time injecting opiates, she was still productive and self-reliant. She described herself as a "*highly functioning addict*", reporting that she would still "*wake up in the morning and go to school and I'd go to TAFE and I'd work*". While addiction explains aspects of Emma's experience, she was very much in control of many aspects of her life and drug use. Felix's use of pharmaceutical opiates also demonstrates a significant exercise of agency while injecting drugs. Felix used these prescription analgesics as a form of improvised medical maintenance, which formed part of a conscious decision to "*get my shit together*".

While self-reliance is a key feature of the way these participants spoke about intravenous opiate use, this sense of responsibility for their own health and social welfare was also often placed within the context of unavoidable circumstances and social marginalization. Emma rejects a complete responsibilization of her transition to intravenous and heroin use, noting how emotional pain at the hands of an abusive partner structured Emma's choices in complex ways: "*[it] sounds really weird, but I was half doing it because um I wanted to get high and half just because I wanted a fucking break from Tom*". When describing his experiences injecting drugs Felix is also critical of the structures that make the lives of people who inject drugs so precarious. In making this criticism, Felix uses the metaphor of opiate use as a fire in a cave. Within the metaphor individual, emotion and social marginalization are like a storm raging just outside the cave: "*And you're trapped in the cave because your wet, and you've got to keep feeding the fire*".

It is also significant to note that participant perspectives made a sharp departure from the kind of individualized self-care promoted in neoliberal discourse. For instance, the need to care for others was an important theme discussed, often brought about by the circumstances of injecting drug use. Emma recalled that, after a frightening encounter with some people who sold her drugs, in which a group of men forced her to use in front of them, those men soon became trusted friends: "*once that happened, they were all very protective of me… Even when I got clean, my main gear dealer came and visited me in rehab. They were really proud of me, really proud*". As noted above, Felix took the notion of peer-to-peer education of harm minimization very seriously. He was active in sharing health information to people new to injecting. Felix showed novice injectors where to acquire sterile equipment, helped them to locate the MSIC and informed them about services related to the transmission of blood-borne infections.

These accounts demonstrate that cultures of injecting drug use structure the agentive capacity of people who inject opiates. While social marginalization encourages self-reliance and harm minimization services certainly can empower people who inject drugs to take control of their health, marginality also encourages care for others who occupy similar life circumstances. The participants' capacity to care for the self and others is, however, inseparable from the conditions of the illicit and precarious street-based cultures of injecting drug use. The capacity to change injecting behavior, avoid overdose, or reduce or change patterns of drug consumption are thus intimately tied to the social context and political economy of their use of pain medications.

As is demonstrated with Felix's example, painkillers can play a very different role in the lives of people who inject drugs than what much of the current literature describes. His account illustrates that an uncritical acceptance of biomedical conceptualizations of 'addiction' may problematically present intravenous and dependent painkiller use, and any subsequent transition to heroin, as representative of practices of non-medical consumption. Empirical examples in previous chapters have already illustrated that there are a broad range of non-medical practices that are in no way limited to intravenous or dependent consumption. Moreover, qualitative analysis of the life histories of people who inject pharmaceutical opiates and heroin can prompt complex questions about how the experience of addiction, and associated notions of individual agency, is constituted at its intersection with structural factors such as gender, class, social history and policy, and medical discourse.

Conclusion

The epidemiological literature about pharmaceutical opiates to heroin transitions record important health information that deserves elaboration, however an overreliance on the psychopharmacological paradigm, risks obscuring the social context in which injecting drug use occurs. Social research perspectives demonstrate that the framework of addiction provides only limited explanations for drug use. Rather than a focus on how drugs impact individual bodies or on how individual psychology impacts choices about drug use, sociologists have instead focused on the structures that shape or produce dependent consumption. In the tradition of such social research, this chapter has argued that drug use is a social practice or experience (Fraser et al. 2014: 3).

For instance, Emma's example demonstrates how gender and class frame the 'addiction' experience (and drug use more generally), while Felix's example illustrates how the stigmatization and criminalization of injecting drug use and addiction can produce individualized appropriations of health and medical practice. Moreover, Emma and Felix are both examples of people for whom there is a life beyond addiction. The idea that people can in fact move on from the 'addict' identity allows for a critical exploration of drug use more open to the sociological imaginary.

This chapter has addressed two key sociological critiques of addiction as it relates to the intravenous use of pharmaceutical opiates. An exploration of epidemiological literature about transitions from licit to illicit opiates highlights the significance of complementary qualitative analysis. The intricacies of transition from and between intravenous opiate use complicate the dominant cultural meaning of licit and illicit drugs. The complexity of the legal status of opiates also calls attention to the political economy of cultures of injecting drug use and how they impact upon intravenous and dependent consumption. Moreover, social science literature about agency in drug use highlights how the choices of people who inject drugs are structured by policy, discourse and personal circumstances.

The conceptual and empirical discussion in this chapter has foregrounded the role of gender and class, the political economy of injecting drug use, neoliberal discourse and harm minimization policy. Understanding how these elements of the use of pharmaceutical opiates intersect constitutes an important tool in thinking beyond 'addiction'.

References

Acker, C. J. (2002). *Creating the American Junkie: Addiction Research in the Classic Era of Narcotic Control*. Baltimore: Johns Hopkins University Press.

Berge, K. H., & Burkle, C. M. (2014). Opioid Overdose: When Good Drugs Break Bad. *Mayo Clinic Proceedings, 89*(4), 437–439.

Blanch, B., Pearson, S., & Haber, P. S. (2014). An Overview of the Patterns of Prescription Opioid Use, Costs and Related Harms in Australia. *British Journal of Clinical Pharmacology, 78*(5), 1159–1166.

Bohnert, A. S. B., Valenstein, M., Bair, M. J., Ganoczy, D., McCarthy, J. F., Ilgen, M. A., et al. (2011). Association Between Opioid Prescribing Patterns and Opioid Overdose-Related Deaths. *Journal of the American Medical Association, 305*(13), 1315–1321.

Bruneau, J., Roy, É., Arruda, N., Zang, G., & Jutras-Aswad, D. (2012). The Rising Prevalence of Prescription Opioid Injection and Its Association with Hepatitis C Incidence Among Street-Drug Users. *Addiction, 107*(7), 1318–1327.

Campbell, N. D., & Ettorre, E. (2011). *Gendered Addiction: The Politics of Drug Treatment in a Neurochemical World*. Basingstoke: Palgrave Macmillan.

Carise, D., Dugosh, K. L., McLellan, A. T., Camilleri, A., Woody, G. E., & Lynch, K. G. (2007). Prescription OxyContin Abuse Among Patients Entering Addiction Treatment. *American Journal of Psychiatry, 164*(11), 1750–1756.

Carlson, R. G., Nahhas, R. W., Martins, S. S., & Daniulaityte, R. (2016). Predictors of Transition to Heroin Use Among Initially Non-Opioid Dependent Illicit Pharmaceutical Opioid Users: A Natural History Study. *Drug Alcohol Dependence, 160,* 127–134.

Carney, M. (2010). *Oxy—The Hidden Epidemic. Four Corners.* Sydney: Australian Broadcasting Corporation.

Cicero, T. J., Ellis, M. S., & Surratt, H. L. (2012). Effect of Abuse-Deterrent Formulation of OxyContin. *New England Journal of Medicine, 367*(2), 187–189.

Chilcoat, H., Abrams, R., Natarajan, S., & Coplan, P. (2014). Changes in Prescriptions of OxyContin and Opana after Introduction of Tamper Resistant Formulations Among Potentially Problematic and Comparator Prescribers. *Drug and Alcohol Dependence, 140,* e33.

Cloward, R. A., & Ohlin, L. E. (1960). *Delinquency and Opportunity: A Theory of Delinquent Gangs.* New York, NY: The Free Press.

Compton, W. M., Jones, C. M., & Baldwin, G. T. (2016). Relationship Between Nonmedical Prescription-Opioid Use and Heroin Use. *New England Journal of Medicine, 374*(2), 154–163.

Dart, R. C., Surratt, H. L., Cicero, T. J., Parrino, M. W., Severtson, G., Becki, B. B., et al. (2015). Trends in Opioid Analgesic Abuse and Mortality in the United States. *New England Journal of Medicine, 372*(3), 241–248.

Degenhardt, L., Black, E., Breen, C., Bruno, R., Kinner, S., Roxburgh, A., et al. (2006). Trends in Morphine Prescriptions, Illicit Morphine Use and Associated Harms Among Regular Injecting Drug Users in Australia. *Drug and Alcohol Review, 25*(5), 403–412.

Degenhardt, L., Dierker, L., Chiu, W. T., Medina-Mora, M. E., Neumark, Y., Sampson, N., et al. (2010). Evaluating the Drug Use "Gateway" Theory using Cross-National Data: Consistency and Associations of the Order of Initiation of Drug Use Among Participants in the WHO World Mental Health Surveys. *Drug and Alcohol Dependence, 108*(1–2), 84–97.

Denzin, N. K. (1987). *The Alcoholic Self.* Beverly Hills, CA: Sage.

Dertadian, G. C., & Maher, L. (2013). From Oxycodone to Heroin: Two Cases of Transitioning Opioid Use in Young Australians. *Drug and Alcohol Review, 33*(1), 102–104.

FitzGerald, J. L., Broad, S., Dare, A., & Foundation, V. H. P. (1999). *Regulating the Street Heroin Market in Fitzroy/Collingwood.* Sydney: Department of Criminology, University of Melbourne.

Foddy, B., & Savulescu, J. (2010). A Liberal Account of Addiction. *Philosophy, Psychiatry & Psychology, 17*(1), 1–22.

Fraser, S. (2004). 'It's Your Life!': Injecting Drug Users, Individual Responsibility and Hepatitis C Prevention. *Health, 8*(2), 199–221.

Fraser, S. (2008). Trauma, Damage and Pleasure: Rethinking Problematic Drug Use. *International Journal of Drug Policy, 19*(5), 410–416.

Fraser, S., & Seear, K. (2013). *Making Disease, Making Citizens: The Politics of Hepatitis C.* Farnham: Ashgate.

Fraser, S., Moore, D., & Keane, H. (2014). *Habits: Remaking Addiction.* Basingstoke: Palgrave Macmillan.

Grau, L. E., Nabarun, D., Harvey, A. P., Irwin, K., Givens, A., Kinzly, M. L., et al. (2007). Illicit Use of Opioids: Is OxyContin® a "Gateway Drug"? *American Journal on Addictions, 16*(3), 166–173.

Johnson, O., & Schardan, R. (2012). The Gateway's Heroin Epidemic. *Journal of Law Enforcement, 2*(1).

Keane, H. (2002). *What's Wrong with Addiction?* Melbourne: Melbourne University Press.

Keane, H. (2003). Critiques of Harm Reduction, Morality and the Promise of Human Rights. *International Journal of Drug Policy, 14*(3), 227–232.

Kolodny, A., Courtwright, D. T., Hwang, C. S., Kreiner, P., Eadie, J. L., Clark, T. W., et al. (2015). The Prescription Opioid and Heroin Crisis: A Public Health Approach to an Epidemic of Addiction. *Annual Review of Public Health, 36*, 559–574.

Kuehn, B. M. (2014). Driven by Prescription Drug Abuse, Heroin Use Increases Among Suburban and Rural Whites. *Journal of the American Medical Association, 312*(2), 118–119.

Lankenau, S. E., Teti, M., Silva, K., Bloom, J. J., Harocopos, A., & Treese, M. (2012). Initiation into Prescription Opioid Misuse Amongst Young Injection Drug Users. *International Journal of Drug Policy, 23*(1), 37–44.

Lenson, D. (1999). *On Drugs.* Minneapolis: University of Minnesota Press.

Levine, H. G. (1978). The Discovery of Addiction: Changing Conceptions of Habitual Drunkenness in America. *Journal of Studies on Alcohol, 39*(1), 143–174.

Lindesmith, A. R. (1938). A Sociological Theory of Drug Addiction. *American Journal of Sociology, 43*(4), 593–613.

Maher, L., & Dertadian, G. (2018). Addiction Classics: Qualitative Research. *Addiction, 113*(1), 167–172.

Mars, S. G., Bourgois, P., Karandinos, G., Montero, F., & Ciccarone, D. (2014). "Every 'Never' I Ever Said Came True": Transitions from Opioid Pills to Heroin Injecting. *International Journal of Drug Policy, 25*(2), 257–266.

Matza, D. (1969). *Becoming Deviant.* Englewood Cliffs, NJ: Prentice-Hall.

McCabe, S. E., West, B. T., Morales, M., Cranford, J. A., & Boyd, C. J. (2007). Does Early Onset of Non-Medical Use of Prescription Drugs Predict Subsequent Prescription Drug Abuse and Dependence? Results from a National Study. *Addiction, 102*(12), 1920–1930.

Meldrum, M. L. (2016). The Ongoing Opioid Prescription Epidemic: Historical Context. *American Journal of Public Health, 106*(8), 1365–1366.

Moore, D. (2004). Governing Street-Based Injecting Drug Users: A Critique of Heroin Overdose Prevention in Australia. *Social Science and Medicine, 59*(7), 1547–1557.

Moore, D., & Fraser, S. (2006). Putting at Risk What We Know: Reflecting on the Drug-Using Subject in Harm Reduction and Its Political Implications. *Social Science and Medicine, 62*(12), 3035–3047.

Nicholas, R., Lee, N., & Roche, A. (2011). *Pharmaceutical Drug Misuse in Australia: Complex Problems, Balanced Responses.* National Centre for Education and Training on Addiction. Adelaide: Flinders University.

Nielsen, S., Larance, B., Bruno, R. B., Lintzeris, N., Vanderhaven, M., Lattas, G., et al. (2015) *Understanding the Health and Service Needs of Diverse Populations of Pharmaceutical Opioid Users: Cohort Studies of Dependent Users in Treatment, and People Who Inject Drugs.* National Drug and Alcohol Research Centre, Technical Report 331.

O'Toole, S., & Connect, P. (2013). *Habit in the English Novel, 1850–1900: Lived Environments, Practices of the Self.* New York: Palgrave Macmillan.

Peavy, M. K., Banta-Green, C. J., Kingston, S., Hanrahan, M., Merrill, J. O., & Coffin, P. O. (2012). "Hooked on" Prescription-Type Opiates Prior to Using Heroin: Results from a Survey of Syringe Exchange Clients. *Journal of Psychoactive Drugs, 44*(3), 259–265.

Pollini, R. A., Banta-Green, C. J., Cuevas-Mota, J., Metzner, M., Teshale, E., & Garfein, R. S. (2011). Problematic Use of Prescription-Type Opioids Prior to Heroin Use Among Young Heroin Injectors. *Substance Abuse and Rehabilitation, 2*(1), 173–180.

Ray, M. B. (1961). The Cycle of Abstinence and Relapse Among Heroin Addicts. *Social Problems, 9*(2), 132–140.

Roxburgh, A., Bruno, R., Larance, B., & Burns, L. (2011). Prescription of Opioid Analgesics and Related Harms in Australia. *Medical Journal of Australia, 195*(5), 280–284.

Roxburgh, A., Hall, W. D., Dobbins, T., Gisev, N., Burns, L., Pearson, S., et al. (2017). Trends in Heroin and Pharmaceutical Opioid Overdose Deaths in Australia. *Drug Alcohol Dependence, 179,* 291–298.

Rudd, R. A., Aleshire, N., Zibbell, J. E., & Gladden, R. M. (2016). Increases in Drug and Opioid Overdose Deaths—United States, 2000–2014. *American Journal of Transplantation, 16*(4), 1323–1327.

Schofferman, J., Fishman, S. M., Harden, R. N., & Kirschner, K. L. (2014). Did We Reach Too Far? The Opioid Epidemic and Chronic Pain. *Physical Medicine and Rehabilitation, 6*(1), 78–84.

Sedgwick, E. K. (1993). *Tendencies*. New York: Routledge.

Vosburg, S. K., Jones, J. D., Manubay, M. J., Ashworth, J. B., Shapiro, D. Y., & Comer, S. D. (2013). A Comparison Among Tapentadol Tamper-Resistant Formulations (TRF) and OxyContin1 (Non-TRF) in Prescription Opioid Abusers. *Addiction, 108*(6), 1095–1106.

Weinberg, D. (2011). Sociological Perspectives on Addiction. *Sociology Compass, 5*(4), 298–310.

Wingood, G. M., DiClemente, R. J., & Raj, A. (2000). Adverse Consequences of Intimate Partner Abuse Among Women in Non-Urban Domestic Violence Shelters. *American Journal of Preventive Medicine, 19*(4), 270–275.

Yokell, M. A., Delgado, M. K., Zaller, N. D., Wang, N., McGowan, S. K., & Green, T. (2014). Presentation of Prescription and Nonprescription Opioid Overdoses to US Emergency Departments. *Journal of the American Medical Association: Internal Medicine, 174*(12), 2034–2037.

Conclusion

While non-medical painkiller use is presented as a form of 'drug abuse' in much research and policy, the findings of this book illustrate that this kind of consumption is not the domain of a deviant or aberrant group characterized by pathology or criminality. Participants in this study derive from diverse backgrounds and lifestyles, including tradesmen and stay-at-home mothers, students and professionals, people with established full-time jobs and people who work on multiple contracts across different industries. Similarly, the motivations for painkiller use across the sample are mixed. They range from use for mild physical discomfort and social anxiety to injecting use and dependent consumption. Contrary to the stereotype of the 'seductive' drug that coaxes its user into a life of dysfunction, this book illustrates that when people use analgesic medications there is an intimate relationship between the motivations of pleasure seeking, health practice and productive citizenship.

The types of use outlined in the book do not exist in a vacuum: context is key. The medicalization of pain and suffering in late capitalist societies has fostered higher public expectations about the therapeutic qualities of pharmaceuticals and medicine's ability to cure and control the body. Higher expectations about therapeutic medicine have

G. C. Dertadian, *A Fine Line*,
https://doi.org/10.1007/978-981-13-1975-4

informed a cultural context that demands a 'pill for every ill'. The development of a pharmaceutical 'pill culture' has also fostered an expanded understanding of pain, as well as the medical promise to alleviate it. These expectations, alongside ideas of preventive self-regulation and self-care, now represent a significant threat to medical authority. The threat that creative medication consumption poses to medical authority appears to be feeding contemporary concerns about non-medical 'abuse'. Yet, a critical assessment of a growing set of research and the analysis of interview data suggest that non-medical consumption may in fact be commonplace and disparate.

This book has contextualized the real and serious harms of prescription opiates by providing a detailed qualitative assessment of the discourses and practices that comprise non-medical consumption of these medications. It has drawn on scholarship about the structure of late-modern society to critically examine a discourse of abuse that has come to characterize official accounts. This involved tracing historical evidence that reflects how concern about the danger and harm of opiates has shifted over time, often related to matters of professional control rather than scientific clarity. The book has traced the social meanings of opiate and analgesic consumption through its legal, medical and political histories. An emphasis on the historicity of the harmful properties of opiates has highlighted the way knowledge about analgesics often conflate a range of levels of drug consumption and exaggerate its relationship with criminality. The book also explored the way medical and commercial discourse shape contemporary understandings of pain, and how pharmaceutical medications are used to manage human suffering. Closely linked to this is the way human experiences of pleasure include the alleviation of human suffering, often in unexpected ways. Participants use painkillers for relief from physical discomfort and find that it this also has affective qualities: it makes them feel productive, numb, and even inebriated.

This conclusion will draw together the key concerns of the book to develop some overarching conclusions about medical authority, neoliberal theory and contemporary understandings of pain and pleasure. The conclusion will also elaborate on some of the implications of the findings for future directions in theory, research and policy.

Medicine and Consumption in the Age of Anxiety

Medical and scientific knowledge have important impacts on the way painkillers are consumed. The work of Foucault has been particular influential in empirical and theoretical analysis of medical knowledge and drug consumption. Foucault argues that knowledge is central to the operation of power, which can be both repressive and productive (Foucault 1980). Medical knowledge does not simply describe self-evident pathologies; rather, it is central to and productive of pathologies related to drug use. This involves both the way medical knowledge informs legal distinctions between kinds of opiates and biomedical discourse about their impact on the human body.

The way medical knowledge informs legal distinctions between kinds of opiates has been a significant theme throughout the book. Part I outlined how the convergence of medical and political knowledge throughout the twentieth century produced and entrenched distinctions between kinds of opiates and the people who consumed them. Political rhetoric addressed and perpetuated concern about the apparent depravity of the hedonistic 'Chinaman' and the vice of urban youth. In response, legal frameworks were produce around drugs like heroin to make them illegal and thus reproduce the idea that they could only cause harm and suffering. At the same time, medical frameworks defined morphine (and later OxyContin) as medical technologies that heal or reduce the suffering of the body. These frameworks inform socially constructed distinctions between the legitimate consumption of pharmaceutical products and the illegitimate consumption of illicit drugs. Such distinctions, between 'legitimate' pharmaceutical consumption and 'illegitimate' illicit drug use, are challenged by the emergent discourse of painkiller abuse.

The medicalization and pharmaceuticalization of work-related-stress is a key empirical example. Physical manifestations of stress affect the productivity of the modern worker, and this has recently been the subject of increased medical intervention. Pharmaceutical companies have sought to capitalize on social anxieties about productivity by presenting pain as an impediment to work—and thus also positioning the consumption of their products as a way to be more productive. Medication users take up aspects of this part-medical-part-commercial ethos by using painkillers to prevent, pre-empt or interrupt discomfort and illness.

Observations about preventative consumption are particularly pertinent in light of social theory's insistence that medical science does not simply articulate preexisting disease states or biomedical facts. Rather medical/scientific knowledge constitutively produces professional understandings of disease and biological realities. This has important impacts on the way people experience the uncertain conditions of modern society. Feelings of anxiety and other emotional responses are thus also medicalized and pharmaceuticalized in a range of ways, involving a specific set of legitimate medical treatments.

As discussed in Chapter 3, the medication of emotional pain has a long history. The most direct type of medical intervention into emotional discomfort came in the form of pharmaceutical tranquilizers ('happy pills' and 'emotional aspirin') during the 1960s. Since the introduction of tranquilizers, medical treatment for social and emotional unease has been expanded to include a wide range of pharmaceuticals such as antidepressant and stimulant medications. However, as examples from this book have illustrated, when medical interventions are not available or do not meet cultural expectations about therapeutic potential, medication consumers appropriate 'legitimate' treatments through creative consumption. In this context, the loss of a loved one, dealing with an abusive partner, and managing the marginalization involved in cultures of injecting drug use become ideal circumstances to appropriate medical discourse and practice.

Critical analysis of medical knowledge is also required to unpack the moralizing imperative of addiction discourse. The medical model has become a prominent way of understanding regular or prolonged drug use. People who use drugs even internalize aspects of the medical model of 'addiction as disease'. While addiction is widely regarded as a genuine biomedical disease in medical literature, this does not necessarily ameliorate the moralistic elements of addiction discourse more generally. Medical practitioners often treat people who use or inject drugs with deep skepticism, significantly impacting the kind of treatment and care on offer. The institutionalization of 'addiction as disease' has been influential in producing drug use as a 'legitimate' medical condition; however, it also informs the lived reality of the 'addict' who is treated as an illegitimate patient and often as not deserving of treatment. Moreover, the conflicted status of the opiate addict in medical treatment is exacerbated by the way painkiller use frequently slips between the categories of legitimate and illegitimate consumption.

The reluctance of many medical professionals to treat people who inject drugs like 'ordinary patients' with a 'legitimate disease' also adds to the fragmented and uncertain circumstances of their everyday lives. This is also compounded by the limited availability of services for drug dependence. The moralization of addiction and the scarcity of services contribute to the way pain medications are used to manage opiate dependence. The use of pharmaceutical opiates to stave off withdrawal is seen as 'safer' and easier to predict. This predictability provides some sense of certainty in precarious circumstances. The use of a pharmaceutical alternative to heroin in order to medically maintain patients has been available in Australia since the 1970s. Conscious use of pharmaceutical opiates to avoid heroin thus represents an acknowledgement of the therapeutic potential of pharmaceutical intervention. It may even be argued that people who inject drugs internalize medical models of drug use, so much so that they appropriate medical treatments like OST when those services are not available or convenient.

The role of medical discourse and power has been a recurring theme throughout this book. Medical discourse constitutes feelings of anxiety about uncertainty as a biomedical reality that has a pharmaceutical solution, it consolidates neoliberal notions of appropriate production and consumption, and it colonizes the common understanding of prolonged drug use as a medical condition—addiction. While people certainly adopt these external structures, they also bend and subvert aspects of medical authority. In this light, non-medical consumption is best thought of as a conditional appropriation rather than a rejection of medical power.

A Note on Neoliberalism

A key element of the way people appropriate medicine when using painkillers non-medically involves individualized modes of consumption that draw from neoliberal ideology. Aspects of this book have thus been devoted to exploring the role of neoliberalism in constituting and shaping practices of non-medical consumption. There are two observations about neoliberalism that can be made when reflecting on the findings of this book; the first is that the emergence of non-medical consumption is further evidence of what we already know about neoliberalism—which is that it encourages the responsibilization of health practice by insisting that the individual (or the medication consumer) holds primary responsibility for their own well-being; the second is that neoliberalism is no longer simply an ideology held by a privileged few in the capitalist class, and imposed upon everyone else without their permission—it is now an intimate part of the way people practice their work, their lives and their leisure.

Historical and conceptual analysis in Part I outlined how neoliberal economic policy has impacted on the provision of social services, and the role this plays in the development of problematic drug use. Part I also explored how a neoliberal focus on the individual can erode support for individuals who are unable to 'take responsibility' of their own health because of structure barriers to do so. This focus on and deferral to the individual is also a key feature of the commercial push for 'self-care', in which pharmaceutical and other industry bodies advocate for an expansion of consumer access to pharmaceutical medications.

Social theory is largely critical of the way neoliberal discourse espouses a-political 'empowerment' of the individual because this does not take into account structural impediments to the accessibility and actionability of knowledge about health. While this book has demonstrated that there are many and various structural impediments to the neoliberal ideal of individual consumers 'freely' managing their own consumption, it also acknowledges that people who use analgesics non-medically take up this kind of individualist discourse. The use of painkillers at work provides a requisite example of how non-medical consumption can be informed by a commercialized imperative for individualism. As noted throughout, people engage in non-medical use in a range of ways at work. Pain from a headache or anxiety over work is met with individual appropriations of already medicalized and pharmaceuticalized processes.

For instance, painkillers are used preemptively to 'bulldoze through' work, respond to stress and manage lack of sleep. The imperative to 'do whatever it takes' to stay healthy is thus connected in important ways to the imperative to 'do whatever it takes' to be a productive (and thus valued) worker. In this context of intense focus on productive work, the medical connotations of pharmaceutical analgesics sometimes feed into consumer rhetoric. The painkiller becomes one product among many on the supermarket shelf that can be used to 'pep you up' and 'keep you going'. Neoliberal discourse thus informs potentially lucrative (and exploitative) notions of the responsibilization of productivity and the freer use of medication in order to manage the flexibility required for modern work.

The relationship between 'working hard' and 'playing hard' is also informed by elements of neoliberal discourse. The imperative to be productive is tied in important ways to forms of commercial consumption that allow the 'release' necessary for the continuation of the capitalist cycle of production and consumption. The consumption of alcohol is thus a significant component of neoliberal and commercial interest in the productivity of the modern worker. Use of painkillers to enhance 'time-out' rituals of alcohol intoxication is a key example of an individualized appropriation of the established and thus legitimate social order. However, as examples in the book have demonstrated, for young people in particular, the influence of the neoliberal imperative for individualism is not restricted to appropriating 'legitimate' forms of consumption.

The use of illicit drugs is also associated with the subversive appeal of forms of 'risky' consumption. Here, it is worth elaborating on and fully conceptualizing the way the 'risks' posed by the unproductive body and recreational consumption is negotiated. Edgework scholars have described how the conditions of late-modernity may encourage risk taking. The ideals of capitalist accumulation are built around 'high-risk' investments and stock market exchanges that produce 'high rewards'.

The domains of commercial sport and leisure increasingly incorporate 'extreme' and 'risky' activities like blood sports and base jumping. For many young people, the appeal of risky behavior is built into the social structures that shape their identity and sense of self. While social conditions produce a demand for productive work and healthy living, as well as excitement and risk taking, the circumstances of modern life rarely meet such expectations. Within criminological literature, men in particular are thought to respond to the relative boredom of their everyday life by defying risk and reveling in the 'danger' of activities like drug use. This is certainly part of the way many young men spoke about recreational consumption with pain medications. Importantly however the notion of 'reveling in risk' also formed a central element of women's response to the pressures of managing both professional and domestic responsibilities. The neoliberal imperative for individualized consumption to remain productive workers and mothers propels women's capacity to revel in risk.

Another key feature of the experiences of the lives of young people in this study is recreational and analgesic drug use as a way to 'escape' everyday life. Literature about the normalization of recreational drug use has noted how young people who use drugs are increasingly treating illicit substances like they would a commercial product: they weigh up the potential harms, cost, social repercussions and possible pleasures to make informed decisions about the consumption of illicit drugs. This is another example of the way neoliberalism has begun to inform social practice related to drug use. The expansion of neoliberal rhetoric may thus also be eroding trust in medical and public health knowledge about drug use, instead shifting the focus onto individual experiences with drugs and their harms.

Instead of heeding public health warnings about the ills of drug use, young people respond to public health concerns about the harms of recreational drug use by using painkillers, or adding painkillers to a combination of recreational drugs. The use of painkillers means they can avoid the dangers of engaging with illicit drug markets and provide certainty around the quality of the drug they are consuming. This means that young people can 'stay safe' while engaging in recreational consumption and that they can do so by circumventing the moralizing and punitive elements of medical and policing approaches to drug use. While a medical practitioner does not, for instance, sanction the use of painkillers to 'come down' from ecstasy, use of analgesics in this way clearly has medical intention.

The examples of non-medical consumption outlined throughout this book demonstrate that people take up elements of neoliberal individualism as a form of self-governance. Medication users take seriously the idea that they are 'rational-choice agents capable of self-government' (O'Malley 2004: 333). Productive capacity and the responsibility to consume are mediated by analgesic consumption through individualized appropriations of medical and health discourse. The imperative to rely on altered forms of medication use is tied to contemporary constructions of productive citizenship and a tendency to defer to the individual to manage the uncertain aspects of modern life. The precariousness of the lives of people who are imbedded in cultures of injecting drug use makes an emphasis on the individual particularly salient. However, these improvisations of consumer and health discourse do not only produce individualized discourses.

While neoliberal individualism helps to produce an imperative for creative medication consumption, there are also collective and social aspects to non-medical consumption. Neoliberal individualism facilitates the establishment of 'new' practices that are subsequently expanded into more collective forms and are distributed through social processes. For instance, analgesic medications are often shared among friends, both to spread the benefit of recreational pleasure and the ability for peers to 'be safe' when using illicit drugs. In cultures of injecting drug use information about how to use medications to alleviate chronic pain, difficult emotions and peer-to-peer education about harm minimization when using pharmaceutical opiates are key ways of managing the lack of stability in such environments.

The examples outlined above are illustrative of a dialectic of neoliberal individualism. Non-medical consumption is neither fully individualized nor completely social. Practices of non-medical consumption involve a constant negotiation between structure and agency. This book discusses instances of neoliberal governance, but it also highlights how non-medical consumption is illustrative of the failures of 'governing at a distance'. That is, the individualizing imperative of neoliberal governance can have unintended consequences that encourage people to be 'enterprising' and 'innovative' (rather than compliant) in their dealings with legal and medical authorities.

Pain and Pleasure

The core theme of this book has been to detail how experiences of pain and pleasure are not separate phenomena, and how practices of non-medical consumption highlight this. Pain can be alleviated through the pursuit of pleasure, and the pursuit of pleasure can have painful consequences. A key element of this observation involves a reconceptualization of pain that has occurred in the medical, social and commercial fields and has been taken up by participants in the study. This section will reflect on the way pain is conceptualized in the late-modern age of anxiety, and the way this informs pleasure and painkiller consumption.

Traditional accounts of physical pain have featured as an important part of how people understand pain and get access to pain medications in the book. A range of study participants consumed medications left over from direct prescriptions related to physically painful conditions. Some participants indicated that they only discovered the intoxicating (and pleasurable) potential of pain medications when simply trying to relieve pain. Moreover, for some participants relief from intense or prolonged physical distress was itself experienced as pleasurable. There are, however, other than physical elements to pain that have been explored throughout the book.

A key element of the reconceptualization of pain outlined has been to recognize the way physical, emotional and social discomfort is governed. Examples throughout have illustrated how pain impedes human interaction and hinders productivity and thus often requires immediate (medical or pharmaceutical) intervention. Under such examples, pain becomes a political and economic category, subject to the governing practices that comprise broad areas of human life: including social interaction, workplace relations and health practice. The structures of late-modern society thus play an integral role in the way pain is experienced and analgesic medications are consumed.

Sociological accounts about the conditions of late-modern society are useful in explaining how social structure can inform experiences of suffering (Bourdieu 1999). Contemporary social theory has described how risk and uncertainty have become central to the modern condition (Beck 1992). Buaman's work in particular is salient for a discussion about the relationship between social conditions, emotional worry and medication consumption. His theorization of liquid modernity describes how contemporary society is 'incurably fragmented and atomised, and so incredibly uncertain and unpredictable' (Bauman 2007: 14). Uncertainty features significantly in interviews with study participants.

One example of the role of uncertainty in medication consumption is the way the stress of working environments or the demands of domesticity impact on physical pain. The book explored how the imperative to take responsibility for others in your care (which often involves paid employment) can have a significant effect on physical (and especially chronic) pain. Stress about financial security and the health and well-being of loved ones can compound physical discomfort and may even impact unexpected flare-ups of chronic pain. These examples demonstrate that physical pain does not exist in a vacuum and that it cannot be separated from the social environment in which it is experienced. In this way, the accounts of physical pain provided in this book support the broad movement toward a biopsychosocial model in pain medicine. Moreover, these examples provide a clear illustration of how pleasure and relief from pain are intimately intertwined. Where the suffering of physical pain is extended to include the way pain impedes sociability or productivity, the removal of barriers to socialization and productivity become enjoyable by comparison: where pain once stopped you from interacting with family and friends or doing your job properly, there is pleasure in being freed from the pain to play with the kids, catch up with friends or do your job well.

Physical discomfort is not, however, the only form of pain discussed in the book. While the specialty of Pain Medicine places emphasis on the role of the social and emotional in the experience of physical pain, the field is largely silent on the issue of social or emotional difficulty being painful in-and-of itself. A small but growing body of scientific research has begun to explore the common neurological responses induced by physical, social and emotional suffering. Many of the empirical examples in this study present important complementary qualitative evidence about the way social conditions and emotional responses are experienced as painful.

Discomfort from stress at work and the way this affects the capacity to work are key examples. Managing the stress of paid employment in the context of accelerated yet increasingly precarious working environments informs feelings of anxiety. In such a context, people use pain medications to help manage stress at work, both in anticipation of physical illness and as a result of discomfort induced by intense worry about work. This is particularly the case for those in part-time and casual employment, who need to be seen as 'always on' to remain appealing to employers in order to secure temporarily renewed or future employment. The addition of educational or domestic responsibility often compounds the demand to flexibly manage financial and social life. These conditions are also gendered in a range of ways. The masculine imperative to demonstrate worth through financial means informs men's anxious use of pain medications to remain productive. While for many women social pressure to both work and care for those dependent on them compounds social and emotional worry about their performance as employees and mothers. For many participants, there is pleasure in the numb feeling that mitigates the pressures of work, family and social life—there is also pleasure in the relief that the numb of the painkiller provides.

Use of drugs to numb oneself from emotional issues has a long tradition in drugs research. Emotional difficulties have long been regarded as a pathway to injecting and dependent drug use. Discussion of the lives of many of the participants in this study builds on established evidence that emotional anguish can inform problematic and dependent drug consumption. In saying so, it is also significant to note that for many people who use drugs, emotional pain and drug dependence cannot be separated. Moreover, the experience of drug dependence can also be thought of as a form of suffering in-and-of itself. Opiate withdrawal is not only physically debilitating but it also reduces people's capacity to participate in society. For instance, opiate withdrawal hinders the capacity of the person experiencing it to attend or 'perform well' in a job interview. The need for immediate relief from the painful and debilitating sting of withdrawal is thus an important feature of the experience of opiate dependence. Just as emotional pain and drug dependence cannot be easily separated, neither can opiate use to alleviate withdrawal and its use for pleasure. While participants who inject pharmaceutical opiates and heroin certainly describe a physical euphoria from use of the drug, they also describe the way they enjoy being able to 'feel normal' once withdrawal is relieved.

Beyond withdrawal, there are also broader social dimensions to the pain of those who become drug dependent, and especially for people who inject drugs. The moralizing implications of addiction discourse can have a transformative effect on the social status and self-concept of those who become drug dependent. Familial and social support tends to fall away when medical practitioners and social networks become aware of injecting and dependent drug use. The lives of people who inject drugs are thus incredibly precarious. Being marginalized from wider society in this way erodes people's self-esteem and can produce painful emotions related to reflections about one's own self-worth. The 'high' of the opiate thus provides more than an enjoyable physical feeling—it also reduces anxiety about the way the user is marginalized, numbs them to the thought that they are ostracized from family and friends and provides the capacity to 'sleep it off'—both psychically and metaphorically.

The contexts outlined in these examples are illustrative of the fragmentation of social relations discussed by social theorists more broadly. Large social institutions such as the nuclear (and supportive) family, scientific medicine and full-time employment are less reliable as foundations of support for vulnerable people. Bauman notes that, under such conditions "all drawings of a line are provisional and temporary, under threat of being redrawn or effaced, and for that reason they provide a natural outlet from the wide range of anxieties born of an insecure life" (Bauman 2007: 80). Medication consumption becomes the answer to anxiety about insecure and uncertain life circumstances. Medical and commercial discourses provide culturally intelligible frameworks for legitimizing people's feelings of anxiety and their consumption of pain medications to alleviate it. Because definitions of pain now include social and emotional discomfort, the pleasure of intoxication is difficult to separate from the amelioration pain—pleasurable inebriation is an unconventional, if not effective form of pain relief. In a world full of painful uncertainty, the pleasant and predictable effects of a pharmaceutical opiate that numbs, provides inebriation or relief from withdrawal becomes a cure-all for the debilitating elements of the modern condition.

Where to from Here

The challenge for further research is to recognize that non-medical use is not simply a matter of unauthorized or defiant consumption. Changing understandings of pain and cultural expectations about the therapeutic potential of pharmaceutical drugs should be brought into the medical and epidemiological literature. A greater emphasis on or recognition of qualitative research would help to complement the clinical focus of the bulk of the current body of research. Qualitative research allows for the self-explanation of those who engage in the practice to form part of how it is understood and disseminated. Further qualitative research is thus needed on the meaning of informal medication sharing and lay care practices, pleasure that is constituted by relief from suffering, and the creative appropriation of medical consumption, so that such consumption is not unnecessarily pathologized and criminalized. This would allow for a fuller picture of the kinds of practices that comprise non-medical consumption, and the most appropriate responses to them.

It is also important for both researchers and policymakers to recognize that non-medical consumption is not a homogenous practice defined by a necessary transition to intravenous use and 'addiction'. As recently as April of 2015, the Australian Medical Association renewed its call for "a real-time record of patient prescriptions amid an alarming rise in doctor shopping and deaths" (Rollins). Supply-side policy approaches, such as the proposed introduction of an ERRCD, borrow heavily from international and domestic policy about illicit drug use. This convergence with illicit drug policy is built on the assumption that non-medical use is pathological, criminal, or both. However, as this book has demonstrated, there are a range of practices that constitute the non-medical use of pain medications and they are by no means limited to 'abusive' or 'addictive' consumption.

Many of the practices discussed in this book reveal as much about the way contemporary society is ordered as they do about the pharmacology of the drug being consumed or the psychology of its consumer. Because non-medical consumption is tied to everyday experiences of productivity, consumerism, legitimate forms of intoxication (with alcohol) and common emotions, it cannot simply be dismissed as unimportant, nor dealt with as though it were congruent to injecting or dependent drug use. The drawing of lines between licit and illicit drugs, pain relief and pleasure seeking, productivity and play, medical and commercial consumption are no longer a relevant way to understand this type of consumption. Assuming that the office or domestic worker, the occasional or recreational drug consumer and the injecting or dependent drug user have the same needs for services should be avoided. Research and policy need to account for more nuance by describing and responding to the range and the complexity of practices that make up non-medical consumption.

References

Bauman, Z. (2007). *Liquid Times: Living in an Age of Uncertainty*. Wiley.

Beck, U. (1992). *Risk Society: Towards a New Modernity*. London, Thousand Oaks, and New Delhi: Sage.

Bourdieu, P. (1999). *The Weight of the World: Social Suffering in Contemporary Society*. Stanford: Stanford University Press.

O'Malley, P., & Valverde, M. (2004). Pleasure, Freedom and Drugs: The Uses of 'Pleasure' in Liberal Governance of Drug and Alcohol Consumption. *Sociology, 38*(1), 25–42.

Rollins, A. (2015). *National System Urgently Needed to Counter Doctor Shopping, Drug Deaths*. Australian Medical Association. Retrieved April 23, from https://ama.com.au/ausmed/national-system-urgently-needed-counter-doctor-shopping-drug-deaths.

Index

G. C. Dertadian, *A Fine Line*,
https://doi.org/10.1007/978-981-13-1975-4

Kolibri 360 GmbH
Ferdinand-Jühlke-Straße 7
99095 Erfurt, Deutschland
produktsicherheit@kolibri360.de